MIND VOICE OF OUR BODY

SELF CURE

M DHANANCHEZHIYAN | POPPU

In the memories of Dr. Fazlur Rahman
MBBS DV MD Ph.D. (Acu)

Contents

PREFACE

This text deals with the Natural Healing of the human body. Which is written with the experienced manner of self-healed. For every health issue, we are in a hurry to go compulsory to the hospital. This will really change your thoughts about health at the end of the book. This text was written in the Tamil language. Tamil is my native language. The Tamil text *en udal en moolathanam* was written in an elegant manner I enjoyed the text which pulled me to translate it to English. The saint Thirumoolar says "Enrich your body, be a healthy soul." From Ancient times to still East Indian People cared more about their Health. Could You find the health after it was LOST?.

This Non-Fiction was written in a Fictional way. You could get easily the Life, Health, Food, and Self-Cure. I have made a Translation for the readers to understand the easy way. I hope you are going to feel what I felt.

with Love
-M. Dhanachezhiyan.

ACKNOWLEDGEMENTS

My Uncountable thank you! to the Notion press which brings this Text to widespread Readers. And I would like to hold the hands of the Orginal Author Poppu Purushothamam has a belief in me and allows me to Translate his work. In every literary work, he was the first reader and critic of it. The translation idea was started with the words of Chandra Sekar Iyya, a Tamil Professor. with such love and support I wish to bring more south Indian writer's work into translation. and a special mention here, Tamil copies were Published by Santhiya Publication a hearty thanks.

POPPU

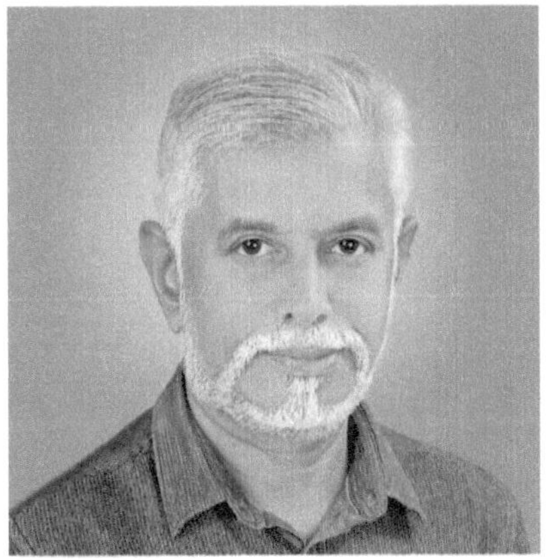

About Author:

Purushothaman @ poppu. Dob 7.3.1960, Birth place - kovilangulam village, 40 km south from madurai. At the age of 14 written poems. In 23 written and staged dramas for social movements. In his thirties started to write short stories. The very first story won state-level awards. Stories published in Kalki, vikatan and literary magazines. Short stories collection published by vikatan publication. Translated around ten books from English to Tamil on environmental, health, social issues, and politics. Wrote essays serials on health and food for three years in Tamil Hindu and malai malar. Ten books on health and food were published by Santhiya Publication. Run healthy food restaurant for ten years at Hosur. Now servicing as an Acupuncture therapist for 12 years. Having clinic at Chennai in Guindy and Vadapalani. And regular visits to Vijayawada, Hyderabad, Nellai, Bangalore, and Selam. Studied ITI Worked in Hosur Ashok Leyland company for ten years. Worked as a technician in Singapore for ten years. kavipoppu@gmail.com

M D

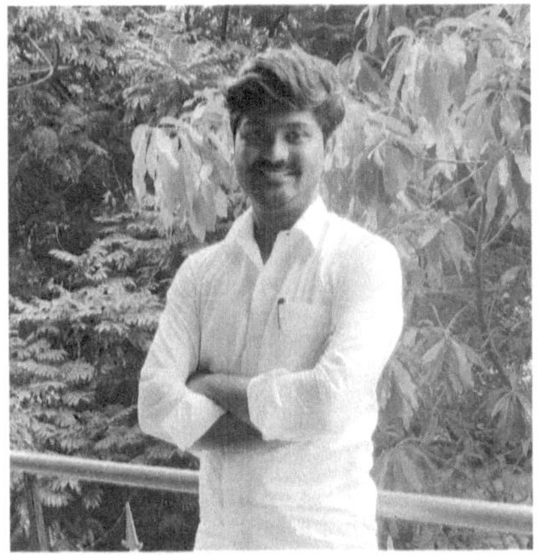

Translator

About Translator:

M Dhananchezhiyan was born on 02 June 1994, in Kovilpatti. He now lives in Chennai, Tamilnadu. He completed his UG in English literature at presidency college, Chennai. And PG in Pachaiyappa's College, Chennai. And working as Assistant Professor, Department of English in Vel Tech Ranga Sanku Arts College, Chennai. He started writing in 2014, he writes bilingual in English and Tamil. Doing translation of Indian Languages. Writing genres are Poetry, Short Story, Essays, and Articles. His Poem, Short Stories, and Articles are published in Print magazines and Online Magazines. Three compilers published his work. He is also an executive committee member of the Tamilnadu Progressive writers artists association - Aram.

dhananchezhiyan.writer@gmail.com

I
Talk to the Body

We chatted with the girlfriend, and we conversed with friends. The cell phone gets offers, and we talk, talk, and keep on talking. From the school, they asked, "Talk to your son then only you know, what the trouble is?" When you get to know that we are doing that consciously. As we are taking responsibility for others' words.

Something new in the working culture. Salary offers, confirm promotions, pretending memos, though it is not enough to increase production and the gain! they are having the everyday meeting, and a weekly meeting as they continue things with the meeting, meeting, and meeting.

From those meetings, they talk until your ears are completely affected by the 'bee…..' sounds.

We prepare well for the meeting and aim to listen well.

As we are not enough with those talks, we started to chat about our private life with the traveller who travels with us on the train. And that makes you feel, you are losing your stress.

We spend more time talking. It was a prolonged thing that we are doing throughout our lifespans. It was calculated Superficially. We spend it as a major job.

Have you talked to your own body? Have you listened to your body?

The body is insisting on something with you daily. Have you felt listening to the body?

From the movement of birth until the last, when something affects our body that is with us. Have you compassionately inquired about that? "What happened to you?"

We inquire about the health of any relatives or friends to give them mental health, and the courage to stay healthy.

But when something happens to our body we take the body to the hospital and leave without any cross-examination. As if we are leaving the vehicle to the mechanic and listening to him.

The mechanic is highly regarded as the Bike Doctor. But, in reality today the body is treated like a machine. What do we say to those who had made the body as a machine?

When something happens to the body. Before lifting it to another person and running away. If you talk to it calmly, it will tell you what happened to it.

We can have a small conversation with the body and solve the problem smoothly. Even international issues solved by talking? Then, why are we rudend to the body?

Rogue treatment is not an ordinary issue. Professional assassins also dare to work that they do not dare to do. The womb is a part of the intestine, and they delicately cut rotten legs and arms in the name of diabetes.

Does, it mean that you have to take pills now and then to cure the disease? Even though taking medicine is not cured!

If an particular disease occurs, it will not be cured. They keep on saying that you have to live with pills all the time, as they are threatening like the school child by snatching money and telling you, "Why don't you go for a walk, sir?"

Not even for physical health. Fearing the doctor's threat, we go for a walk. It doesn't even work after a walk. So, does this regular walk make sense?

Walking is not something useless; the drug after the walk is useless. And it doesn't make any sense. It makes the disease permanent in the body. And spent a lot of money on it. And it manipulates the disease in the body, as we say in the medical term "Side Effects!"

As they have taught us to accept the Side effects.

If there is no use of drugs as you want to do walking and some more exercise. As if there are also side effects. Then, What is the use of medicines?

In the beginning, We drank alcohol for ecstasy. Later we drank because of the effects of being drunk. So what is the difference between medicine and alcohol? It becomes more respectable when We spend more on medicine than alcohol.

Let us see a simple example.

Today's morning when you get up and pee which is not in a regular pass. Urinary incontinence does not occur even after passing four to five times. Even after trying it doesn't work.

We return to bed. No one else in the house has woken up yet.

We're just getting used to thinking. So, the thinking has evolved. If our thinking goes above and beyond it is not self-thinking.

Thoughts cling to one or two things heard through the neighbourhood, newspaper, and television. We are in our thirty-five. In the middle of the age Some uneven diseases occurred. (Such a thought is injected into your head before it occurs) and they convince us that diseases come naturally as we are aged.

Look at how good thinking is. We too are running out of family, children, duty, and responsibility all the time without ever looking at the time. So anything can happen to our body at any minute.

What is the problem if the pee does not pass properly? What is urinary incontinence? Kidney. If so, there is a problem with the kidneys.

That was supposed not to drink alcohol Saturn. But when it comes to a party, a tour, and enjoyment with friends when friends and superiors are persuaded we can't avoid it.

What to do: We have all been born good children since birth. (they told me I was so good) Could you change that habit from now on?

Even so, liquor is not so regular. somewhat like, twice or thrice in a month. Even so, What do they blend with? those who combine something with the infant's milk. How could it not combine with liquor?

Why unnecessary thinking for this? No matter what happens to the body, it is better to see a doctor immediately and find out what is going on and get it fixed on the pills at an early stage. Otherwise, the problem behind will be to face many problems such as operation, insurance, leave, and job change.

Why? even life...

"Damn, Chandru, why do you think so?"

"Looking around. Three lives dependent on us are sleeping peacefully. What will they do if we do not?"

"Wipe your tears, Chandru. You should be brave. They are holding up their minds." said the Doc.

Is it possible to trust doctors these days? Everything has become a business. so you are going to Dr Mohan very close to you.

He might be a doctor but, Mohan is your friend?

He praises your sense of urgency and refers to Muralitharan, who is close to him, saying, "I'm not a kidney doctor!"

When Mohan rejects. There is tension in Chandru. After grabbing him with two, or three phone calls he got an appointment. Chandru is scheduled to see urologist Muralitharan this evening.

As he was thinking about this, he did not seem to notice how it was urinating. After the morning. Is it a regular pass? Did it have any difficulties?

We don't remember when we last urinated. This is how we rush without remembering what we are doing. That makes us unable to pay attention to physical well-being. Then, you are making for a chance to go to the restroom.

It was less. No pain or irritation. Now comes the second idea of whether to look at Dr Muralitharan

You are asking an office colleague. He says a lot more about it. Muralitharan. "It was lucky to get his appointment. Go and check. Happy if it is nothing.

It cost around only five hundred. (lives are just five hundred.) If had an infection, a kidney stone or a problem with the bladder means that would be better for the health to know in the beginning"

He wasn't concerned about the kidney so didn't want to waste the appointment with the Urologist Dr Muralitharan, a urinary specialist. He went to him.

Needless to say, what is going to happen there, here are a hundred experiences for many people.

The fact that the urine did not pass as a regular form and that the intellectual questions and answers bubbled up inside you was 'greasy and slippery'. A sense of duty and concern for the family arose. You talked to the doctor. You asked a friend for advice.

But you forgot something important.

What's so important about it? Is everything alright?

What is more important than concern about the dysfunction of the body; concerning someone randomly and wasting time and money; more than abusing the self element; What could be more important than getting an appointment with a specialist doctor who cares about the body and cares about it?

Let us see if it is right or wrong. Let all this be on the side. All the activities you took care of took place outside of the body.

That action must take place within the body if the dysfunction is to be resolved. You make no effort for that.

You started thinking, Will it be an infection? Is it a kidney stone? Want to see a specialist? Have to be on long leave? You are afraid that they will be robbed of a lot of money.

The body that has cooperated with your life for so many years without any major problem then what right now? you do not believe that nothing will happen.

Did we sleep properly? Did we eat anything that should not be eaten? Were we in a colder or hotter environment? So, is there a chance of a change in the pass of urination? Have you had a urinary problem before? You haven't cross-examine yourself as to how cured it is.

Our ancestors spent a lifetime enjoying life without taking pills and without seeing a doctor for a long time. We never thought we would get such an opportunity.

Not only is there a urinary problem that we have now. There may be a hundred reasons why we have physical illness.

It does not have to be complicated. After thinking for a long time that the only way to solve it is to see a doctor and take a pill, don't suddenly conclude.

There are so many opportunities. Urinary incontinence can also be cured by taking a bath with an extra bucket of water in the morning. Let it be cured in a tumbler of hot water. Half a day of rest can be. Can be fixed in tender coconut. Or the days may last.

At least there is no mental opportunity to notice how the urine is passing next time. Excessive tension.

Our people will say a proverb: "don't be in a hurry. Everything arises in a due time"

A scene comes to mind.

We are Indians. The elephant can be seen as ubiquitous. Elephants are rare animals in many parts of the world except in South Asia and Africa.

The elephant trunk, which weighs fifteen tons, can even pick up a sewing pin lying on the ground.

The elephant's eye is capable of seeing objects beyond two kilometres. The elephant's ear is capable of hearing sounds that occur five to eight kilometres away. The elephant has the power to smell what is there. Not to mention its physical strength.

Such an elephant obeys the order of the circus master and rings the neck bell. Similarly, many people in the outside world go to the doctor and shake their heads.

We believe that the doctor knows everything that we don't know about our bodies. The reason is that if we talk to our body, then only we learn about the physical. We never spoke.

The one who thinks he has big companies in his hands and the one who rules the country. Were been shaking the bell in front of the doctors like the elephant in the circus.

What else can be done?

What if something happens to the body without listening to the doctor? Who will protect my family? Who runs this company? Until my son studies. I should be alive with this physic?

I alone spare the 'EMI' on all the products I buy? Questions like this were screwing like an arrow on you.

Do nothing else, Talk to the body for some time.

How can you talk to the body?

II

The silent melody is sung by the Body

How to talk to the body? What does it talk to us about? We talk to pets. What does the Kitten and the Mischief Dog talk to us about? Do they know any language? Understand, what we are saying in the use of our voice. Do, we understand its moans and groans?

Did the girlfriend who recognized your first love speak any words? She showed a twinkle in her eye. How is it that only you out of ten understand that it is an expression of love for you?

The Boss is sitting behind a desk, looking between the forehead and the frame down to the nose. What does that mean? "You go and come after some time?" How could I understand what was saying with his eyes without saying, Why did you return quietly?

The moment you turn the key in the vehicle, your wife wipes her wet hand in front of you, realizing that she's standing with a request for something, and you seem to ask, "Tell me."

As when you know so much? Do you not understand what your own body says?

Have you not made such an attempt yet? It's okay. From now on, after bathing, ask your body, "how is it now?"

It will say. "What is so cool! everything is now bright to the eye."

Dinner at a friend's house. You wander and get tired. Good appetite. Friends and wife waiting for you "Just sit there. Let's have dinner." The body cooperates for your civilization even when you have a good appetite. You ask gladly. " It's okay, I will have it later. Have you all eaten?"

Five minutes later you sit in front of the Banana leaf. No matter how hungry you are, listen to a word to the body without causally moving your fingers towards your favorite ingredient. Ask the Body "What can I eat first?"

Though the energy drained out. The body will get happy first as you ask. It says "dessert"

If the stomach is a bit dull. The body will be preferably too spicy.

Well, now you taste the dessert. The cells of the body are all Renaissance. You are hungry and eager to taste. The stomach appears to be overeating as it is empty. You ask the body "Is it Enough!" when it reaches the normal level!

Then, the stomach will say "Okay, Enough, and Stop!.."

Instead of asking about enough, what about a little more? if then the stomach will say "OK, let's eat a little more."

Our body is like a mother. The mother will conform to the mind of the child. Eventually, she will struggle to carry all the burdens on her own. The body bears the same until it bears and suffers.

We need a precautionary sense that our body should not be harmed in the same way that a mother can be tolerated if her child suffers.

The body can adapt to our sense of alertness. That's what talking to the body is all about.

The body is always giving small signals. Taking care of them and fulfilling the needs of the body will compensate for our tendency to the end without causing us great inconvenience.

For example, you went out and ate with friends this afternoon. You continue to work in the office. Is mildly tired.

Regular tea time. Beeps with a little bad smell. You ask yourself,

"What the hell?"

"Aha! Let's leave. Shouldn't it be like this for a while? Why always have the tongue and mouth under control?"

The answer is not always to be in stiff control. There is nothing wrong with going out with friends and having all that stuff. But.., but. Now you are not in a healthy physical condition.

In this environment, everyone is going to drink tea. Did not seem to drink tea. Why even seem to have difficulty in walking? It's like dizziness. (Body sings a silent tune) You say to friends, "You go and have."

Feelings of guilt over letting you alone. They ask, "Although Nothing, let's have tea."

You comply with their insistence. It looks like the faint was better now.

What is happening in the body now?

Showing his discomfort. The body is begging you. "Look here, Chandru. the lentil powder and ghee at lunch. It's more than usual. Then be like chronic lentil powder. Had a lot of ghee. I accumulated all my strength and digested it. That's when I signaled a stinky. Beyond that when you got up I showed slight dizziness. Beyond that, you went and drank tea. You belong to us. What do you do? What should I do now? Although I have not yet digested what you ate for lunch, I set it aside and for now, I am starting to work on digesting this tea. what else to do?"

The body sets aside the digestion of lunch to one side. Such stagnant waste is just waiting for the opportunity to emerge.

If Chandru would have gone for a long walk in the evening or the night before or beyond the city bustle. Most of the accumulated waste will be cleaned. Or you may be starving instead of eating that night. Or if you have eaten fruit Or fruit juice as a portion of simple food, the body will have restored to normal.

Ancestors have followed this strategy. We, who are accustomed to the mechanical approach, try to find a medical solution by treating the body as a machine. We think of resolving the crisis that has occurred within us within our body from the outside.

Does not understand the silent melody of the body. Not talking to the body.

We often talk to our conscience.

When making an important decision. When there is a commotion.

Fighting with the wife for trivial matters and being in a stage of resolve.

Dominating The children and feeling guilty.

Conscience asks us, "Did the eight-year-old boy do something unknown?

Is it wrong? How could you dominate him? The child is swelling"

"It is wrong! Then how could he learn?"

"What does it mean? You have the right to beat the child! isn't it anarchy that even one's child beats? Teach them patiently. It's the beauty of teaching. If you do not have the patience to teach, you will not be able to have a child.

"Once or twice how many times I have been telling to him, there is no point of shouting at all"

"When your father beats you, do you think he was right? Or when he taught at first, did you do well?"

We have been talking to our conscience so many times. Did we learn by ourselves to speak with conscience, or did we learn by watching an image emerge from the character in the films of the seventies and stand-alone and speak?

Somehow we are talking to conscience.

Similarly, we need to talk to our bodies.

Only if it speaks to us do we speak to it.

The body is always talking to us. We do not listen.

Do not ask when the body spoke, like the Parasakti verse "When the idol of God spoke" It's always talking. What we have lost is the ability to hear it.

If the body speaks out of the mouth you will not bear it. That is why it speaks a silent language with pity on us. Whatever the consequence, Isn't a body?

It, therefore, tries to make us feel as much as possible without harassing us. It raises the rhythmic sound only in the mature state.

Many of us snore in our sleep. "Zzzzz,...Srnkk...." Watch out for others snoring. Not even five or six times does the same constant sound. The reason is that the maintenance work of the body is going on so hard and so fast. The body urgently needs the breath of life.

To compensate for the body's request, the nose, the respiratory organ, and the lungs, the body's internal organs that purify the air, attempt to inhale air as a matter of urgency.

Because the nose and trachea (and oesophagus) are not clean enough. Dinner and the fat stored in the abdomen for a long time clogs the space required for the lungs so that the body is not able to get the air it needs.

As there is not enough air going through the nose, the body opens its mouth and breathes for its own needs. The body draws air through the nostrils for a while, then through the other nostrils for a while, and then through the nostrils for a while. So that the noise drawn by the wind is not constant.

On days of heavy snoring, when you wake up in the morning, your throat, mouth, and nose are dry. Snoring not only dries the throat but also causes the chronic upper jaw extremities to bulge forward. Worn tooth, The lips twitching, The face becomes deformed. The reason for this change is not aging as many people think. The feet are the result of abdominal heaviness.

We can see that some people are getting beautiful even with age. The body of such people can often be seen to be lite without being tight.

What does this snoring, dryness, and facial expression mean to us?

Keep the airway clear. Give enough space to the lungs and keep the weight under control.

The human race does not snore until the end of adolescence or until the age of 23 (or) 24 when the body's growth is almost complete. Animals other than humans do not snore.

It is only when physical abuse increases, when symmetry decreases, that the body even raises the snoring sound. Otherwise, it wants to be light in its course.

If we begin to pay attention to the signals that the body arouses when the body's symmetry decreases, we will understand what it means.

For that, we must always have a conversation with the body.

III

Talking to the body

Before going to bed at night? As soon as you wake up in the morning or in the middle of work? When is the best time to talk to it?

Your body is not something alone behind a huge table in a room. It is not sitten with supremacy in a reclining chair wrapped in a turkey towel up to the neck.

You do not need to get an appointment for it.

It is with you.

To talk with that, there is nothing scheduled like what monarch makes, you can talk to it always.

The body may have been angry staring at you at some point. May have liked the contradiction. May have been inconsistent. Despite all this, it did most of the time cooperate.

So, you start talking to it without looking at any arrogance. It will continue to express its will, opposition, consent, and denial. You can change your habits accordingly. It will prepare itself as you like. There is no better way to be healthy than to have body and soul working together.

Chandru Your age is 35. You have to pick up a one-kilo file from a table three feet away from where you are standing and place it on the table three feet away on the right. Suppose you take forty files without your mental will. Severe pain can occur in both your shoulders.

But you go to the gym with the desire to keep your body fit and start at twenty kilos to weigh fifty to sixty kilos. Now you will feel the pain in your shoulder. Over time, that pain will go away. How is it?.

There is a mutual understanding between you and your body. The body adapts to our mental desires.

At no age does it cause unnecessary harassment. Just like stuffing the cotton into a pillow, we're just pushing the strain into our body and harassing it, saying, "nothing has been adopted."

Look at our ancestors who lived in the villages about twenty or thirty years ago. Until a year or two before dying, they had worked in the woods and relaxed a little. And end up.

"How was the granny?"

"Better now! Speaks well, but it couldn't take food."

What? no food. It is hard to get over until the dark moon, That might end soon. It's hard. But, anyway. He deeply possessed all the wealth. Nothing was left. Call out the grandchildren, she might watch out and die with peace of mind.

The lives of many parted knowingly. It shook hands and said

'Goodbye' without any difficulty to the body where it was staying.

But today, Many deaths occur just as said, " I was never aware of it. he was so good until yesterday."

A man with no cash on hand and no regular income. He is not even comfortable putting petrol in a patch-up vehicle. Suddenly, I didn't know magic could happen. He built a new house. There are individual vehicles parked at the house.

He is roaming everywhere. He was good until the morning.

When it was difficult to breathe, and sweating. The ambulance arrives with a threatening shout, "Waaaaaaahhhhhh..., Waaaaahhhhh...." the cart with two brave men goes to the hospital.

The doctors said, "Well, you're on time. There is nothing to say if it was an hour late. No need to be afraid now. It needs to be operated immediately. Once you pay for the whole package.

For the particular days offering the cots and foods and plan to stay there. Is It a vacation?

Healthy body matter is considered as a package means, who filthy it is. But, it doesn't make sense to us.

We are paying three or four lakhs immediately. Those who are asking for the urgency of operation, are neglecting it now because the body condition is not getting ready. They scroll out the days

Then the operation takes place on an auspicious day. Loved ones are all waiting outside the theatre with trembling hearts.

The doctor arrives and wipes his hands with a Pale white turkey towel that smells like a hitherto unknown scent.

He is the one who has spoken to us many times. Now we see his face that he will say something to us. He passes by without noticing us. We are going behind. He looks at us with the question, "What?"

We tell the doctor who underwent the operation that it is relative to us. "None of you should disturb him," he warns. (oh god! Gives anesthesia and makes it look like a corpse, cuts with a knife, and takes things out. Sews it like a corner bag and puts it on the bed. How anyone could disturb him more than you.)

When the last drop of the energy is absorbed. The body has no choice but to lie down one day and recover itself.

We need to pay attention to the rhythm of the body.

As we give attention to the bank balance after swiping the money at the ATM.

When you are forcing the body into machines, as the health advisers say, and waiting like a beggar for the doctor's response to a paper that was given by the laboratories are shameful activities.

We must be masters of ourselves, at least physically. We come from the outside. There is someone new in the house. His presence is uncomfortable for you and the families. Will you bruxism your teeth and stop talking?

A friend comes to the house and asks who the newcomer is. "I don't know. He has been here for the past two days. Can't tell this man to leave the house. I do not know what to do?"

He tells a good idea. "Would you go to the police station and complain? What does it mean not to take any steps?"

"That means to spend a thousand or two thousand rupees on a police case."

"Don't worry about all those, if something is wrong to happen how could you be with that? Should be get rid of it." Are we going to get to this point?

You know, How to evict someone who has entered our home unnecessarily without the advice of others or the cooperation of the police. Similarly, our body does not need any rude medicine to remove the illness.

In the same way, we are to be the masters of our bodies. We must prepare ourselves according to the will of the body. Body language can only be understood by constantly interacting with it.

When to talk to the body? How to talk?

Speak up every night before going to bed, says naturalist 'Lindler'.

Think about the body, What it has been doing After Waking up this morning. How did it cooperate to do all the work?

After the lights are off, stare at the ceiling and don't think about unwanted things. we should conduct inquiries as to whether it is necessary. What foods did we have? What is in them for the taste of the tongue? What is in the best interest of the body? (They both are the same. These distinctions will automatically disappear when it comes to the right lifestyle.)

Depression can affect the body to any extent. It has become unavoidable to this day. If such a situation arises tomorrow we must conclude that it should be avoided.

How far have we progressed towards a lifestyle that is in harmony with the body and nature every day? To what extent were we compatible with the love of fellow beings? That should be taken into account.

"Whenever I saw a withered crop, I withered," said Vallar.

There are no ancient songs that do not sing about nature, animals, landscapes, the world, and the rain. Our Batton Valluvan, who has adopted a morality that should be followed by all the people of the world, concludes our first song with 'primal world'.

A Versifier worthy of admiration with any other poet in the world

He begins his song with "Everything in the World".

With such immense traditional pride, we must cross-examine ourselves every day to what extent we live as children of nature. This cross-examination begins with talking to the body.

Let's do this every day before going to bed, as naturalist Lindler says. But, when are we going to start talking to the body?

Let's close this page at this moment and start talking to the body right now.

IV
How to Talk to the Body?

Don't want to swallow saliva. Don't want to strike up. Nor is it not preparation for proposing your first love.

Let's start abruptly.

"Sorry. I haven't spoken to you ever."

The body is closer to you than anyone else in this world, so it begins to talk to you with a loving sign by putting a hand on your shoulder.

"It's okay, you aren't in the amendment or Egoed not to talk with me. Since I have been near to you that makes you want to talk later. Now you have the sense to talk. That's the happiest. then?"

"Haven't I spoken to you yet? So I do not know what to say."

"Accurately, well the beginning would be like that. Then, day by day, the two of us would not be able to stop talking."

"What You're is right. We'll start talking first. It would be nice to begin talking from a message that suits you."

"Yep! Tell me what suits me?"

"You're a bit of a jerk today. You're like wind, you're going to be able to run like that."

"It's okay. Good. As soon as you noticed me, and realized I was light. Joyous"

"Thanks. Did you tell me the reason why you are lighter today? Can I follow it regularly?"

"I don't want to be lengthy. I said things straightforwardly. What did you eat last night?"

"What yesterday night? Night? Oh! No, I haven't taken anything. It's a lot of work and tension throughout the day. It was irritating yesterday. So, I took a bit of a break and leaned on the sofa, forgot everything, and slept without having supper. Haven't woken up in the middle either.

"Correct. Haven't taken anything. I'm so much better."

"What? It is quite confusing to me. I have heard that not having food will make you weak. But, you are quite the opposite of that. And says you're better now."

"Yeah, all the elements of the body have become weak from the course of your work and the tension you had yesterday. I could not have digested the item even if you had eaten it that night. Fortunately, you did not eat. I am relieved. For the time being, I did not need energy through food. Everything in the viscera needed to be adjusted. There will always be an energy reserve. You do not have to worry about that."

"Throughout the day the excess acids secreted by the body were ejected. And I ejected the rest into the urine. And make the pinched nerves normal. Now I'm better. If you would have taken an additional idly today. Although I wouldn't trouble you. I will put it in Reserve Energy. I will make up for the excess that spend on last night. Don't Worry! Be Happy."

"We won't die. If you haven't eaten for the day" I heard Shivaji say in the movie The Gold Medal. It is new to know. If we haven't taken food for the night. It will be easy for you to do the maintenance work. And you will be lighter then."

"Might be New Or Old. It is lighter Right."

"Yeah, there is lightness"

"Then, don't worry dude"

"What a joke it is not to eat. It is not difficult. It's time saved from eating, and Money Saved. Dear Bodie, But then you will run out of energy. you're going to suffer a lot."

"I too don't have difficulty. It's you. You can't be without food for a certain day. Habitual is not able to be defeated. If you have not eaten, I will clean every morbid inside you and I will keep everything perfectly. Then when you get down to work I will support you with Energetic.

If you have not eaten for years. I will not let you die. It's not a compulsion to have food for a living. The energy within me. When you exit the limit by hard work, it should be given back. I will warn you of any palpitations, faintness, etc. Otherwise, if you are not working and not having anything means also I won't leave the soul out. My body is not a rental house for your soul. The body is the Own house for the Soul. Only if I have secured the soul I too can secure myself. If I send the soul out. The next day a worm came and started eating me. That is why I will not give up your life for the sake of not having a normal meal. You're just thinking of something unwanted."

" Hey look, don't make fun of me. I'm not eating for the taste bud. I'm having food, the body of you to get energy. "

"Then what? Have you ever asked me before having anything? You wish to eat whenever you like! Taking three idlis in a hurry so as not to miss the bus, I was putting the bath experience into mind. There you are moving out of the bathroom. When I'm not hungry, the idlis that you are taking are falling like stones. When I am trying to digest the Idil there, you are running to get the bus. So, I stopped digesting and ran for you with full energy to get the bus.

Are you allowing me to do anything completely? When you are going on a bike before a turn, is it used to indicate with an indicator and used to show your hands as a single? That's good too. But, have you ever indicated anything to me before taking any action?"

"Can't get you?"

"Can't realise. Okay, I will tell you as we are concerned about each other. When I'm in the way of something, you are diverting me onto something. Is it confusing or not?"

For example, when you are looking at an account that has not been tallied, your manager comes and says, "Chandru, come with me quickly, we need to go to the bank." What would you do?

"I will say, Sir, in ten minutes I will finish this account and we go, sir."

What if he says, "No, come with me now."

You will get irritated and angry.

Yeah, the Same I get. You would like to take a rest by not being sleepless and watching TV until twelve. And you get to sleep in the early morning, while there I use to regenerate the dead cells. There the alarm rings and you wake up before I complete You thought in mind not to be lazy and move fast. then what happens all along the day I feel sleepy. And you will say with boredom, "What the hell to this body feeling sleepy."

Ok, let that go, then after waking up while taking a bath the heat is not properly dispelled. While in the bath you get to remember your friend's housewarming. So you started soon from there. What the hell are you doing? Your wife may get angry so you take the coffee without thinking about its taste and temperature. And before I get ready you pour the hot thing into me and move to your friend's housewarming. With tension, you have something there before the coffee gets digested. Then you move from there to the office. I keep on exploiting the adrenal gland for your anxiety."

"How could it exist with adrenal acid instead of blood? How far can I compensate? There are acids which regulate your body although, To relax on weekends you are consuming alcohol. What could I do?"

"Oh! Well, now I can understand your situation."

"It's not enough for you to say only, yes! If you tell me and do anything I will compensate for your behaviour, if not?"

"Okay, let it be like that from now on. Tell me what to do, and when to do it, and I will continue to do so. If you become a rough cow, then I will be feeble."

The body thinks as it taps the right corner of the forehead with its finger.

"'what a thought?"

"Nope, Since I have been speaking plainly for so long, I am thinking that I can also speak a little more openly and unhesitatingly. Only then will we get a clear solution to our problem."

"Hey, what are you saying about the problem? I can't handle it already. What else are you doing to scare me?"

"Look here. Is it a problem? It's become a habit for people to run away and think about it. I'm telling you that I can find a solution. Then why are you afraid? If you listen to me, I will be useful to you."

"You are the only body I have. You always stuff with me. Oaky tell what it is."

"Brother. Don't get bored. Where would you go without me? As I leave you poor. If I put it down. You know I'll never rise again.

"Okay, well I talked to you too in the habit of talking to everyone. Unsolicited. Tell me what to do. I will continue to follow."

"Mm, then you're ok with this. I'm asking for your concern."

"That's what I'm Surrendering, Then what?"

"Okay, Come I will say, Whatever you decide to do, do it completely.

Don't think of unwanted things while travelling, and Do not talk unnecessarily while eating. Don't wash your hands halfway through an urgent call without knowing whether you have eaten or not. Don't have concerns for others which I don't like. Don't do anything to make me suffer. I said I want a good sleep. Who spares time for anyone... Do you spare some time daily for me who is with you?

"What do you want to do to have time with you?"

"I have run so much for family, earning, work, and friends. I'm the only one who compensates for all the purpose, dear, spend some worthwhile time with me."

"Spend some time?"

"Don't worry. Set aside twenty minutes. We can both talk and walk for a while. Settle the account for the respective day. Prepare for the next day. Every day can be trouble-free."

"What a thought. Why aren't you responding?"

"Nothing, I wonder if I can go walking for Daily."

"What can be done if it can't happen? But if you make a habit of making time for me daily, talking to me, walking with me, then I will regularise you. If you help me once, I will help you twice. OK?

"You are explaining it naturally, how could I overrule it?"

"Can it be overridden? No problem now. Tell me what other way we can work together."

"No, you are right. Make time for one Make daily. Conducting an investigation. From now on I will only do what you like."

"Give me your hand. Good boy. Even if you make a small change in your daily life until you take a shower every morning and sleep. I will not trouble you till the last minute."

"Thank you so much!, body"

V

Bath until colder

We dirt, aren't we taking baths daily?

we are handling the heavenly in an unashamedly way Saying, "Wait for two minutes I put some water on me and come"

But is bathing just about washing the body? We should ask that as a question.

Valluvan Batton says, "sleep is like death; waking is like birth from it."

How one starts each day. Before opening the shop, the shopkeeper starts the shop only after scratching the shutter as "Tara Tara" and putting a multiplication mark.

Even if the customer is waiting for a business of one lakh rupees, he leaves him aside and puts the joss stick in front of God and shows all the merchandise and only then shows a smiling face to the customer.

Look at a car driver, he warms up and prays, puts combustion camphor in front of the car, and leaves it, puts lemons on the four wheels, touches the steering wheel, and bows, and only after that does he turn the key. The engine whines like a familiar pet.

Why? Even our Chandru before taking the bike to go to the office touches the handlebar and gives a kiss "Mm...ch..." and kicks the kicker.

Do we, who so sanctify everything, adore the body which is the source of all these? Do we take a divine bath to start the day?

Until thirty years ago, it was our custom to bathe in open water that infused this cosmic energy in rivers, ponds, and wells.

After walking in search of the state of water and bowing to it, we will drown in the water and wake up out of breath. A few minutes of breath-holding every day is a health practice. It happened automatically.

While bathing in a state of water the body is soaked for fifteen to twenty minutes. At that time all the previous day's heat in the body is completely cooled down and goes out. The body prepares the heat anew for the bathing day.

The day begins anew. The body absorbs the energy of open water. Today, no water can be seen in the open except for the sewer water.

The rivers where we and brothers and sisters, aunts and uncles fell for hours in all the months of the year, are today just rocks and bones as the sand robbers scooped up the sand.

On the other side, they are also blasting the rock. (Sagayam sir, look here too)

Even if there is no water flowing in any river, the bridges across all the rivers are running heavily due to the help of foreign loans. But it is the silent cries that arise when crossing them that last for a long time.

Since the river is too far away, let's stop talking about the river and come to the water.

At present, the water we bathe and drink in overhead tanks, and underground tanks and cans have become regular users.

After drinking river water and preserving lake water for a day or two, and tasting the water we have now, we can realise how big a difference there is. It is possible to accurately distinguish between the vitality of the ci-devant and the decay of the latter.

Open water is the life energy of the universe that it holds within itself and can provide stimulus, activity, and immunity to man. Filled water can only function with inactivity.

It is an inescapable law of nature.

Our forefathers have experienced and written down. What is the nature of river water, and what are the characteristics of spring water? What diseases can be cured by using well water and What energy the lake water can provide to our body?

Such water was once available in all areas. Today the commonality of water has been taken away. Water is the property of the rich. They kept the water in separate bottles as mineral water. Is there a more obscene scene in our time?

Here, while talking about bathing, we have to talk about water.

It is not just moisture that our body needs from the water while bathing. The energy of the flow of water, the energy of the sun attracted by the water, and the energy of the universe are all.

Our body needs more than just the minerals and trace elements that are said to be found in commercial water. There are many microbial nutrients that our body needs that are not visible to any studies and research.

These bottles and advertisements cannot give away. We have a natural trait, the body will produce all the micronutrients it needs.

So those who live near state water should make it possible to bathe in it two or three times a week.

When going on tours, you should plan an itinerary for the bathing spots.

(On a trip with five friends, we had to stay one night in a town called Kambam surrounded by mountains on three sides. We excitedly talked about going to Suruli Waterfall, which is twenty kilometres away from there. In the morning, the two of us could not be woken up. When we are getting near the cascade the ice scent makes Moving legs a little slower. In the end, I have not said anything about it because it would be bragging if I was the only one who bathed in the cold flowing water that felt like electrifying the body. Completely erase the letters in these brackets)

Places like Okkenakkal, Courtallam, Thiruparappu, Kaveri, etc. should be included in our travel list which is a treat for the mind and body as well as a treat for the eyes and tongue.

Not only do you have to make a travel list, but you also have to take a bath to wash off the body's annual waste three times per destination.

Listen to what your body says after taking such a bath.

Breathing will be free. Breathing is as smooth as a single vehicle plying the road on strike. Legs urge to walk while standing and urge to run while walking. If running. Running is like flying. So bathing is very important for health.

My sister's house is in Musiri. Even after all this, Cauvery water is flowing like a flag for many months of the year. Whenever I go to my sister's house, I never fail to go to the banks of the Cauvery or Mukkombu.

My brother-in-law and his children would bathe with me there for hours and then my brother-in-law would say, "Honestly, I will never fail to take a bath in the Cauvery, it feels young, uncle."

But he will dip himself in Cauvery next time I go there. I keep thinking about whether I should move to Musiri itself for him, for me, and for the savour river fish available in that town.

Those who bathe in tap water daily should take a long bath in open water whenever possible. Bathing at home should not be considered as the completion of the day.

Bathing at night before eating or two hours after eating before going to bed will give good results to the body to reduce the heat rising in the body due to our

work and food digestion, and to relax the tight muscles and nerves, and tension we get from the work till evening,

Night sleep is especially deep. There is no nightmare. Bathing is not just about getting rid of dirt and grime. If these are someone, those who are not dirty and those who are in a cold environment do not need to bathe.

Everyone needs a bath to remove dead cells from the body.

People who are completely in the natural environment, breathe completely clean air, eat natural food without cooking, and do not suffer from any mental stress, do not need to take a bath.

That is why the people of the mountains who are close to the natural environment do not bathe. Does not eat regularly by keeping track of time. They do not follow any other rules of common dwellers. But they live a full life of one hundred and twenty, hundred and forty years without disease. Because they are very energetic.

If the hill people don't bathe then their body cells don't die? In all living things, cells are dying and new cells are being produced.

A body that doesn't follow a regular bath routine finds another way to get rid of dead cells, other than bathing.

I am intimately familiar with the hilly people who live in the nearby hilly areas of Bettamugilalam, Ukkatti, and Anchetty, about forty kilometers from Hosur.

We were asked the usual question "How are you? Have you eaten?" there

won't answer. There is no habit of sitting down and eating as a family by lighting the stove on certain rules. There is no habit of eating so many times a day.

They eat what is available in nature like fruits, honey, tubers, pods and edible leaves. They buy grains like ragi with the money they get from selling the mountain products available in the respective seasons to the traders (the highest sign of merciless looting culture given to them by the traders) and share it with everyone for a few days only.

Some, Charitable Organisations and camps run on behalf of the Government, if a stove is lit somewhere, people who are ten or twelve kilometers away will come with the smell of smoke. What they eat then is the food of the people of the plains with rice porridge. Otherwise, their food is only what nature provides. Some days, even after wandering so far, there is nothing to eat. Regardless of the disturbance, they will go back without showing any rejection.

This is not the place to talk about their way of life and the interference of power in the name of forest conservation. I have no intention of sanctifying their lives.

People who do not eat something called food in the understanding of civilized people end up living a full life. Hair does not turn grey so quickly. Bald heads are rare among hill people. The reason is the energy of nature.

The food of the mountain people was mentioned here to show that the body gets energy naturally when food is not forced into the body. But we have come far away from nature and it is essential to take a bath to restore the body to its normal state.

As mentioned earlier, not only dirt, dead skin, and dead cells are removed, but also the heat of the body is reduced in the bath. In addition, body waste is also removed. Also, the micronutrients in the water are absorbed through the skin.

So, instead of pouring a bucket of water into the bath, you have to bathe feeling that all the heat of the body has subsided. In addition, the body should be immersed in water for a few minutes to attract the micro-energy of the water.

How to know that the heat of the body has subsided?

Herein is the importance of talking with the body. If you observe the body calmly, you can feel whether the heat is still there or has completely subsided.

You can feel the presence of heat by examining the body whether there is still heat or not and by touching the armpits, the legs, and the lower part of the stomach.

Is this possible every day in this time of emergency world? A question may arise for some. Within a day or two, we can feel that the extra ten minutes we spend in the bathroom can add hours of energy to our day.

Especially on a day of physical ailments. When we have shoulder pain, back pain, mild fever, etc., if we take a longer bath than usual, we can feel that the physical ailment is gone as soon as we get out of the bathroom.

It is enough to take a bath for a little more time than usual and reduce the heat of the body if there is no disturbance in the body.

If there is any abnormal disturbance then bathing can be done as a treatment along with naturopathic treatment.

The treatment we are referring to here is not unnatural medicine. We call healing the healing power of the body that goes on inside. If we do these bathing methods even when the body is not bothered, we can feel that the body is healthy and the skin is shiny and moist.

VI

Health baths

I hope that by now the way of bathing, quality soap, honest soap, and healthy soap are out of your mind.

People who bathe in rivers, lakes, or well water according to our traditional method do not need to follow the method suggested here. The method of bathing recommended here is very helpful to those who bathe in the inactive waters of city life.

On the one hand, milk contains calcium, which is good for bones, and on the other side, naturalists say that milk is a white poison. Let this be. What we mean is that milk becomes a difficult food to digest after the age of three due to changes in the digestive organs.

It is not true that "A cup of tea is active" as many people say.

"Then, why man? The number of tea drinkers is increasing even after tea which used to be ten paise has become ten rupees today. Take whatever you want from me. But don't just pluck the tea." as many people have said.

Although I'm a Tea lover too.

It is true that when tea and coffee are drunk hot, the heat causes a temporary enervation in the body. But in the end what it leaves in the body is a state of lethargy, which can be realised if one observes the body calmly.

Moreover, we do not take the astringent taste that our body needs. So our tongue keeps searching again and again at certain times. It is a physiological fact that the body produces an astringent taste even when one does not drink tea. But the body will make the astringent that is easily available to it. That is why tea is a drink that is consumed over and over again.

"Oops! just like if I take a tea, the next line will move"

What we are emphasizing is that milk indolence aside, most of the milk available in the market today is not nutritious, straight from cow milk or buffalo's milk.

As milk production has declined and demand for milk has increased, more than half of milk is sold everywhere, including in Gujarat, which is at the forefront of the white revolution, is powdered milk.

Well, let's say for the sake of argument that there is no powdered milk. Even then this packet of milk is not of good quality.

It is said that the milk advertised on TV as being milked directly from our villages contains various flours for thickening, chemical compounds to prevent the milk from spoiling, foaming foam, and detergent mixed to dilute the contained milk in water. All this seems to be true when you look at the reaction after drinking the milk.

There is a sanctity attached to milk, so when it comes to talking about the use of milk, so many warning lights need to be put on.

Milk pouring is performed daily to the deities. Ayyanar and Madan, who stand with axes in hand and protect the common people on the banks of the lake and in the town limits, do not care about all this.

They all eat the sun, drink the rain, and tear the wind. These Deities are amazingly powerful. Because these are the ones who stand and digest the cosmic energy of the open space.

On the day of the Heros film, for the banner, the milk is poured packet by packet. On the other hand, they pour beer.

In the midst of all this, why don't we use milk?

Don't fall into the fantasy of anointing and wasting it.

50ml of milk is enough. Pour it into a cup. Just like applying oil to the body for a bath, take the milk and apply evenly from the top of the hair to the soles of the feet and leave it for ten minutes, the milk will be absorbed by the skin. Bathing after drying the rest of the body and the heat will make the upper skin of the body shiny. It also feels cold inside.

Good quality milk is also a good stain remover. People who have a sacred image of milk in their minds may have a cognitive block in using milk for bathing. A good alternative for such people is coconut milk.

Grind a half-shelled coconut into powder or grind it into a small jar without heating it and apply the paste from head to toe, let it dry for ten minutes and come out of the shower and you will swear that the world is a cool thing. It will be that much cooler.

In the same jar, strain the coconut milk and drink, and after grinding five or six hibiscus leaves with the leftover, rub it all over the body and take a bath, it will be pleasant to the eyes. The hair looks beautiful and bouncy.

Coconut bathing holds an important place in the culture of the Maharashtrian people of Maharashtra. Their coconut milk method may sound like a disgusting one. But they do it as a ritual out of respect.

If the grandparents or mother and father are going to the daughter's house after her marriage. They prepare a big feast for them, chew a coconut well, take it with milk and bathe it as a sacred duty. If you bathe like that, it means that you have married me(her) to a good worthy place.

Even if we don't go that far, making a habit of drinking coconut milk and bathing with coconut milk can be beneficial for health.

Oil baths are now less. This is especially important in an environment where the use of coconut in cooking is shrinking due to the commercial threat of sugar fats.

Especially after jogging, we can directly feel the boost of running legs and feet by drinking coconut milk. At times like this, if we can calmly have a conversation with the body without thinking about the next task in a hurry, we don't need to take time to go jogging next time.

Really?

Yes, the body automatically takes you to jog.

Ok back to the bath.

Just like eating non-veg for a certain number of days is a habit, eating fruits should be changed into a diet. Then we can understand that we are moving far away from medicine and approaching health.

The reason for this interruption while talking about bathing is that if you get into the habit of eating fruits, the peel of the fruit can be used for bathing.

We can soak the skin of Pomegranate, orange, Mosambi, and Papaya fruits in the bath water overnight and rub it on the body in the morning and take a bath. Or you can grind it in a mixer and take a bath. And too soaking the skins of fruits like Red Plantain, and Plantain Banana(Nendram)

Now liquid soaps and creams with such fruity scents have hit the market. Soap is better than buying them in a hurry. Because these liquid soaps and creams contain chemicals and the fruity fragrance itself is synthetic. We cannot feel the freshness we claim in them.

Gram and MMung bean flour are now used in the bath. Although this may be necessary for soap use, soaking a handful of the Gram overnight and grinding it in a mixer in the morning, and taking a bath will give you even more benefits.

While these pulses are soaking, add a small lump of almond resin and grind them together to make the paste easier to apply to the body and provide additional benefits.

You can soak neem resin and moringa resin in a sequence of almond resin and knead it or grind it in a mixer and apply and take a bath. It can be used by adding water liberally.

Neem resin is beneficial for people suffering from dehydration and dry skin.

Moringa resin is also beneficial for people with nervous problems. The Moringa tree exudes a generous amount of resin. If you take about fifty grams and soak it in a cup, it can be used for a week.

Similarly, when taking a bath with Tulsi, Mint, Neem, etc. in Summer, the water will provide more chillness.

All the above bathing methods may seem expensive and luxurious. But when you consider the health benefits it offers, it becomes very affordable.

Every bath should be performed as a ritual. Self-esteem is not just self-love or selfishness. It can be interpreted that we start from our body to finish anything with care and mental strength.

Now every Middle class builds a bathtub with pride while building a house. But it is just being used as a laundry basket.

One of the natural remedies I have learned is to soak the body in cold and warm water. When the lower abdomen and spinal cord are soaked in water for a long time, there is a complete solution to many health problems.

I went to a friend's housewarming. He was shown each portion and taken to the bathroom. Seeing that there was a bathtub, I expressed my happiness and said, "It's okay, you have built a bathtub with prior thought."

"Nope man! I don't have any ideas. The engineer who designed this house was forced to build it. Where do we get enough water to the bathtub," he said.

That is true. But I told him that if we soak our body in water once a week, we can feel the abdomen lighten and the spinal cord gets stronger.

In this era of increasing joint pain problems and back pain problems, we can solve many problems if we take care of our bath instead of walking to the hospital and testing labs, keeping what we should not keep and selling what we should not sell.

The final and grandest mention of the bath here is the rainwater bath. Let aside the benefits of rainwater. What a great joy to get wet in the rain.

When It's rainy, our parents reach out to their children. They act so responsibly to prevent themselves from enjoying themselves in the rain.

We trust someone and pay money to buy fresh water and drink it. But we have a mistrust of rainwater. A commercial advertises that children will get cold when it rains. Market business and medicine show a great tendency to make nature our enemy.

What is wrong with rain water... Is there anything more sacred than rainwater? Grandy Valluvan said that "rainwater is an elixir."

Let's cheer for Grandy with a statue. But let's not listen to Grandy's words.

Rainwater that can cleanse all dirty hearts is bad for the body. How absurd that the rainwater that washes away all the scum of the town gives us fever.

During the rainy season, a great sadness came over me. I got soaked in the pouring rain for about a week and dissolved that sorrow.

It was a grief that followed until the last breath of life, but there was no better way to save my life than the rain at that time.

Whenever it rains, I take my vehicle and leave. From city roads to country roads to waterlogged roads, I roam around with the excitement of a child.

As if it was not enough to get wet till then when I'm back to the house, I put my head back in the rain gutter. Which feels like waterfalls.

On the smooth balcony in front of our first-floor house, we can watch our three children play without listening to my wife's calls. At the peak of their enjoyment, you can also play with them.

Being drenched in rainwater to the point where the whole body gets cold and the teeth tremble out does not cause any harm to the body. Not only is there no downside, but there are a lot of benefits.

We can identify each of the sweat pores of the skin individually. Eyes will light up. What else, you will have to spend thousands and travel to Kutralam and Okkanakkal to get the bliss of showering in rainwater. Every drop of rain is better than gold.

we don't get frequent rainy showers, the aforementioned bathing methods should be followed whenever possible.

We should treat bathing like meditation. When rubbing the above-mentioned flour, resin and fruit peel on the body, one should close the eyes and not rub it one by one, but rub it with each part after examining it.

When we see a hand that has lost its little finger in an accident, the sense of its emptiness makes us feel relieved when we look at our little finger.

While taking a bath, while applying. "my little finger, How many times have you put a dot on my keyboard with the series that the paragraph extends? Thank you very much. You are the one who stood before me when I wished in every salutation. It was you who put the last morsel of food in my mouth. Will I forget you." say.

Looking at the little toe. "Aha, you look like a cute little chick. why You are like a bullied innocent child? What's up sweetie, the shoes hurting you?" ask like that and relax.

Your heart will thank you if you do. A nerve tingles in the nape of the neck.

Every part of the body is important in some way. This body did not land in a factory where individual parts were locked and finally carted off. At the same time in the uterus, a smooth formation was formed. Body parts develop uniformly after birth.

This is why each part has its place in the body. Otherwise, what is the need for all the elements to continually in every birth for so many millions of years? Isn't it dry and flaky? Every little part of our body is worth admiring.

Not for cutting edge as commercial medical geniuses say.

When those close to us die, it seems that we should die too. This life is so sensitive. But we dare to lose a part of ourselves out of fear of medical intimidation.

Take a look at the nails that grow and fall off. They shine like the eyes of our beloved.

VII

There is no better friend than walking.

We live in an age where we are too lazy to walk to the street corner of a store. Car for family trips. Bike to office. A 125cc bike to keep things on the bike while going to town.

After all the EMI we closed down for vehicles. We intend to get Scooty for shopping purposes, so we started a loan again from someone saying we bought a treadmill and proudly used it like a new broom. Then in a few days, it also becomes an accessory for hanging clothes.

Walking is not just for the legs. It is the path to deep breathing, expanding the mind, seeing the edge of the sky, widening the horizons of knowledge, and so many benefits yet to be discovered.

Modern business makes people spend tens of thousands on walking. and they teach walking knee-jerkly to walk.

Even if we leave for walking, our well-being and bring us shoes. To buy that, They put a bill of one thousand five hundred for that. Walkers in those shoes look down on barefoot walkers like me who aim to gain ground energy.

No trousers, no tracksuit, no shoes for walking. What the hell are you doing? What if you don't walk? They watch us like we are insulting the walker.

What are they don't? watch it like that! Or is it just an illusion that appeared to me?

Well then, why make even a simple walk an expense?

Shouldn't walking simply be free?

If you get down and don't need shoes, they still show you the sandals with polka dots. Their dotted sandals will not give you the good experience that our earth and stone do.

Nowadays, Nothing is left as normal.

Walking around listening to music with earphones in your ears. If you create a friendly circle for walking and keep talking to them, the feet will adapt to the walk. We were adapted to it.

It is a blissful experience to walk alone with bare feet in the open air without keeping track of time. Every part of the body feels comfortable for us. At first, it appears that only the feet are walking. This feeling can be experienced as the movement starts from the stomach and the stomach goes down slightly. When tasting on the tongue, as the vital minerals do. the body gets the same pleasure as when walking and running.

A woman gets even more pleasure when the baby rolls around in her stomach and when the baby is breastfed. You can take my life right now if I am born as a woman to get these pleasures and make men lust after my body.

We walk on the temple stone. Let our feet and the stone smoothed by millions of feet over the centuries speak in secret. Don't our feet have that, right?

Look at the foot shape, our body weighs sixty kilos, eighty kilos, is five and a half feet tall and is one and a half feet wide (don't check if it's correct. Always being researched) Not even a quarter square foot. These feet have been held up to us for so long. It never asked "you are carrying lots of weight. What have you done to me?"

Look at the toddler running towards the street. The children are running toward the outside world without any ambition for dirt, dust, and germs. We drag them into a cage, instil fear into their heads that never existed before, and put invisible hard wires around them.

I had brought my three-year-old daughter to India. who lived in Singai and never set foot on the soil. The day after we got here we were standing on the third floor of the apartment building looking out at the street and talking. A lorry of mud dumped in front of a house for repair work caught her eye.

She said that she wants to go to that land and play. The child had never seen such a pile of sand before. Where did the child who had never seen others play in the soil get the motivation to play in it?

It must have been the genetics that had stirred in her through the ages.

Understanding her desire, I became her playmate and we used to play all the things I knew like "find the stick, House Building, cook Idli" until she got bored.

When the middle-class eyes of the neighbours looked at us playing in the sand like that, "weird" and their mouths murmured, the movements remained unchanged in me.

We never leave children free like that. We have hastily heaped responsibilities on their heads. We suppress it by saying, "Get married soon, you will control yourself."

After carrying all the burdens and the physical stress and mental stress have increased, if we can even walk freely in the way recommended by all the world's medicine with one voice, it is not even simple.

About a hundred years ago, the Torah, Rahul Sankrityayan and many social sages who approached humanity with motherhood wrote that there is no health beyond walking. They said a long hike without any protection was necessary for life to heal.

I have never seen a man like a writer Sundara Ramaswamy listening with the ear in a way that arouses the interest of telling us. I have to say here only what he said about the way to put a dam on his memories about him.

He was about seventy years old when we were delivering that speech. (He passed away two or three years after that) We were walking through the green forest on a wet tarpaulin like an elephant's back. He said, "I can walk twenty kilometres without stopping. So much so that I was sick and weak most of the time at an age when I should have been healthy."

There is written evidence that he was ill. I could not keep up with his pace and realised that he was a man who could walk twenty kilometres.

A friend of mine. My name is Ravikumar. He has a good income in four or five ways like Wholesale drugs, house rental, auto rental, and finance. The beauty is that he smartly handles every business.

He speaks quietly. Which means quietly, and our restaurant boys laughed off too. He would say two words and laugh at everyone and leave.

Every year he goes to Sabarimala for Mount Hosur on foot. He would only take small amounts of money, and two clothes. They don't rent rooms for overnight stays on the way. In the bitter cold, he would wrap himself in a black blanket and continue his journey. He takes the available almsgiving and eats and continues to walk. Where it is not available, he eats in simple restaurants and pushes cart shops.

When asked what made him undertake this Monk trek despite the financial means, his answer was surprising. Increased respect for him.

"Every month I have many lakhs as profit. All the business was inherited through my father. I will continue this until he dies.

I intend to use this income after his death to do useful social work. But due to my involvement in business and handling of money, there is a possibility that this ambition will dissolve with time without my knowledge.

I said to the family to go to Sabarimala Hill for two months in a year and live as a Monk. So I can understand the people, this life and the poverty of most of the people in this country. The plan I have is getting stronger and stronger in me," he said. I have lost contact with Ravikumar now. I don't know if he's a bit of a freak in his goal or not. Now and then I wonder if a man of money has at least such ambition.

Forty minutes of daily walking is necessary at least for physical health, if not for higher life ambitions.

People who browse the web and YouTube for hours every day get bored with "no time for walking."

Any time except 10 AM to 4 PM when the sun is hot is the best time for walking. Can't find forty minutes of it? If all else fails, try walking after reducing your sleep by half an hour. The deep sleep gained from walking will compensate for such reduced sleep time. Even if you spend 500 or 1000 for such a deep sleep, you will not get it.

I was working in a big factory when I started walking. Its work culture was to the point of sleeping during the day. One day when I woke up like that, all I could see was yellow. That lasted for three to four minutes and then became normal.

Intuition kicked in that I was about to get something serious like jaundice. From then on, I would finish my work by three-thirty, giving up on that day's sleep. The horn for the end of the working hours will be blown at four-thirty. From three-thirty to four-thirty, I started walking on the tree-lined road of that big factory.

A walk in search of material cannot be credited to the account of health, apart from a walk that takes place separately for the sake of the body. Some make peace with the hectic rush to catch the bus as a story of "flog to the dead horse". It's all a fake game.

A big shot called me for his health advice. A big shot is not his wealth but his size. Abdominal circumference. If you want to see him completely, you have to go around like the Navagraha while going to the temple.

Well, it only takes five minutes to see a man completely and let's leave it at that. It is not difficult for us to move around when a single person is carrying such an outsized body.

I told him to walk.

"That's what you say. I never fail to walk for forty minutes every day. Walk by walk. I saw many professionals, who were known and unknown. I will walk there talking to ten to fifteen people," he said proudly

I said, "It's all a joke. You have to talk to your body and walk," he looked at me as a tough teacher and looked weird

Did I say something new? Or he doesn't get it? Or what this little thing speaks a lot? I don't understand whether he saw it that way.

Take time alone for physical health. Where to find time for that?

As we walk, we get everything as a matter of course.

Concerning our bodies, we should take forty minutes of walking and jogging every day. Our feet should completely feel the soil.

When the feet touch the soil, our body receives the energies of the earth, the magnetic energy and the solar energy attracted by the earth. The body relaxes to walk. Blood pressure and depression do not occur if the body is relaxed.

We can feel that the morbid water and morbid gases accumulated in the body are exiting out by themselves. If we run to sprout the sweat, the skin will be rejuvenated. Each organ begins to feel its place in its fullness and begins to make sense to us.

As the body becomes lighter, so does the mind.

Ten years ago, when I was doing a huge money-making business, I had to work every part of my body from 5:30 in the morning till I slept at midnight.

During that period, I would suddenly go to an outstation to relax my mind once a month. Staying in the simplest single room available is just a walk away. Or trekking.

On one such trip, I went to Okkenakal in the evening by bike. I went off-season. At night, only fried fish was available for my hunger.

Being a fish lover, I just ate fish without researching its origin.

Usually, I have supper before it gets dark. On that day, I ate the fish fried in reused oil a century ago.

Every day I woke up at five in the morning and went for a walk. On that day Couldn't get down the stairs of the hostel. The body is tight and suffers from Severe back pain.

I went down the road telling my body that I can't let you stay in pain like that. The legs are begging. "Honestly, I can't. As I walked for your wish before but I can't today." The legs begged for the pity of any narrow-minded person who could accept that.

I said, "Right, right... I'm not going to walk in the usual way. But legs, do me one favour. In this town, tiny and large rivers are running around. As we came this far and don't get wet in water and soil, you will never regret it. So..."

The legs came down slightly "So....?"

"Nothing but, there is a river full of sand under that bridge. Let's go till there."

"Then After"

"I don't want anything else. we can go and return as soon as you get dirt on the feet." I said.

"Son, you will not be subdued. I'm sorry I can't. I'm still holding on. I will walk as much as I can. If I can't do it, I'll give it up. To die somewhere in the dust. This morning, there are no people for help at this time," said Legs.

I begged with them and slowly dragged them with my feet rubbing the ground.

"There is a stone. I will go there and sit for two minutes and take a rest."

"Mm....Mm.... Do something. Evil head."

Legs and I sat.

"Here, there is a tree looks closer, Let's go there and take a rest for a while'"

The legs, which were shaking in anger, did not answer. Who left for that?

I sat down under the tree root and pressed my legs.

"Oh...sir, what are you doing?" said legs

I covered the distance of one hundred metres in twenty minutes. As we got down into the river, the legs were looking at me.

They have done something ugly here. Everything that has been set foot here is not included in the calculation. we can return when my feet are buried in good sand." I said.

We went another fifty metres. The morning light was starting to break through the snow.

Another fifty metres to a rock outcropping. I circled it and walked. The conversation between me and my legs is over. Now the back started talking to me.

I could feel the blood running on my back as I walked with my feet buried in the sand. I was walking in a slightly straight position of the body till now and slowly started to walk upright. The space between the steps increased.

The sun arose suddenly. It will be at 7 o'clock. Even if it is hot in that area, it will be cold for up to ten. I walked briskly in the cold. The whole body has become lighter.

Body pains like death two hours ago. back pain. leg pain Now I know where everything went. If you look closely, you can see that all those pains are falling like dust on the path I have passed and on the tracks that I am walking now.

Walking drove away all the pain.

There is no better health friend than walking.

VIII

What kind of sewage tank is the body?

Chandru leaves his bike at the bike stand in the morning and picks it up when he returns home in the evening. Even the carriage standing under that safe shed the bike is full of dust, dust, and smoke. Someone has written an emergency phone number on that dust.

Only after wiping it can the bike be taken. To that extent, the region is full of dust. Dust is the medium that transmits sunlight to the earth. The size and density of dust vary slightly from place to place.

All of us breathe the dusty air that fills this region. What happens to the lungs if the dust from a parked car enters our body? Does the body become? Don't panic.

If so, does the nose of the air inlet have security to stop the dust? Or is it blocked by some filter, nothing? The body does not allow harmful dust near itself. The body has such power. That is why we are alive after all this pollution.

Not only can the dust not enter the nose, but the radiation emitted from the skin stops the dust beyond the body.

The body naturally does not allow the body to get rid of unwanted and harmful substances. It keeps excreting wastes from the food we eat like belching, faeces, urine, sweat and phlegm.

During the day we eat and work, so we cannot use the toilet. During sleep, all the internal organs take full breath and eliminate waste. They kill old cells and regenerate new cells.

Even after all this waste works, the accumulated waste in the body is not eliminated. A little stagnant here and there.

A portion of the accumulated mucus is coughed up and sneezes out. Moreover, once in four to five months or once in a year, the body engages in a total combustion process, creating a fever.

Fever is the festival of Bhogi (festival of burning waste) that the body celebrates.

There is no need to be afraid of fever or to search for a doctor claiming that medicine is magic. Let's say a beautiful proverb. That which came to the head went with the turban. Fever is such a turban.

If you say "fever, I have eaten anything for two days," the answer will be "Are you mad? Why don't you eat?"

Not two days, three days. Even if you don't eat for four or five days during a fever, nothing will happen. In other words, it is better not to eat. The mouth is bitter because of not eating.

The body cannot do digestive work when internal combustion is going on. That is why the body rejects food. That is the reason why many people vomit.

Consuming food during fever is like switching on the main switch while the electricity board is doing maintenance work. There will be serious consequences.

It is because we do not understand what the body is telling us. We impose something and stop the process of waste combustion called fever from completing.

If we get a fever, instead of celebrating it, we don't give the body the rest it needs, we take a pill and leave the office as if the earth would stop if we lay down. As a result waste disposal does not take place completely.

The waste that should now be burned and expelled is kept in a corner by the body.

Waste that is not expelled in a cold, waste that is not burned in fever is like a pawned jewel coming to auction with interest. More dangerous than colds and flu, the waste is manifested in various ways like jaundice, appendicitis, kidney stone, pain in the spine, and swelling of the knee.

Even now, we give enough rest and eat nutritious food to stimulate the body. Instead of giving the waste a chance to leave the body, we put painkillers and nutritional pills and compress them inside.

What does the body do next? Accumulates waste into cancerous tumours. Or it tries to induce paralysis and hasten the elimination of waste.

It wants to try to stop the brain function and put it in a coma and eliminate the waste.

When common people are lying in a coma, their organs are harvested in the name of organ donation, stopping the traffic and putting the city in panic and transplanting them into the bodies of wealthy patients in big private hospitals. They kill comatose civilians.

Well, that's organ donation. If someone in power, a very rich person falls into a coma and is declared brain dead, they will harvest his organ and transplant it to a common man who needs it in a public hospital. Then the ambulance will 'yink' 'yink' and fly from there to here in eight minutes? Have any of us asked this question?

We know all the cases of them being kept in comas and brain dead as they say for years. They kept him as a minister and not just a patient.

Back to waste.

Commercial medicine admits that the accumulation of waste in the body is the root cause of disease. Commercial medicine also knows that when waste goes away, the disease goes away. Glucose is loaded immediately for any disease. It is part of emergency waste disposal. A transient boost occurs when glucose is loaded. Even when the patient sits up, they bring the lab report in hand and threaten you to pay money by threatening to give you the same treatment as they say "you have this, that?"

Commercial medicine acknowledges the concept of waste stagnation but does not tell people.

Commercial medicine, which loads people with all kinds of medical jargon like cholesterol, sugar, bp, ebola, and Sunana, does not pronounce the simple word "waste removal" to the people.

When the accumulated wastes are removed from the body, the disease will disappear without the help of any medicine.

This is a very simple theory. If the knowledge about waste disposal becomes widespread among the people, there will be no jobs for medicine, drug sales, specialist, fly-in operations and sending patients like Singapore to America.

People who test their sugar after eating and increase the level, take millions of sugar tests and give people digital meters in their hands and create a mental brand of being a patient. "Sugar is gone." Have you at least once made a happy announcement, "Dum dum dum sugar gone in urine"

People called sugar high. Take pills, and take insulin. Have you ever had the word sugar is normal and told you to take it easy?

If they pass the age of 40, they make people wait for the disease whether it will come today or tomorrow, Or the next day.

Even if we don't go to the hospital. Normally people can't stand it if they are excited. They come to the place where four people gather and do a free check-up and write a piece of paper saying "one has that, one has this, the fat is too much. come to the hospital and pay for it", stuff it in their hand, and leave. Just keeping that paper on our head is enough to keep us awake all night, and even if we do sleep, we will have bad dreams and we will become a patient of Sadzad.

I don't know how they recognize us. They hold them like a chicken and make them a permanent patient.

By 2025, India has set a target of making half of India's population diabetic.

The body never wants to harbour disease within itself. Just as a fly sweeps away the dust on its feet the moment it sits still, just as a honey bee beats its wings six hundred times a minute, it makes great efforts to remove any disease from itself.

So much dangerous waste is kept aside on one side of the body and the most dangerous waste is expelled in its course without any notice of pain.

Just as our respiratory function never rests even for a single minute throughout our lifetime, so does our waste elimination function never rest even for a second.

The reason is that the energies of air, water, and food entering our bodies are impure. We cannot measure the amount and nature of cosmic energy that our body receives. But it is unlikely to be impure.

monks (not counting pot-bellied Vedatharis) refuse food, refuse water and seek only air and cosmic energy to think. They sit in meditation outside where there is pure air and in the beginning, they try to get rid of all the waste from the body by getting only the energy of pure air. Then they hold their breath. They suppress the flow of thought. By ceasing thought and breath, they want to give up their own body and merge with the universe, making their life energy universal and omnipresent. They want to penetrate every living being.

So a sage is not the only one who has renounced domestic life. He renounced everything for himself, devotees, monastery, food, clothes, air, and thought. One who finally expels life from his body and wants to merge into the universe. He who thinks that is bliss. Let us not indulge in an unnecessary inquiry into those who claim to be wise, and those who make others say so.

What we are saying here is that our body will retain waste until we stop breathing air. We cannot all become sages saying that we are going to eliminate waste. We don't want greed for happiness.

Let's try to reduce the amount of waste accumulated in the body and reduce the burden of diseases until we die naturally.

Waste accumulates in our body in two ways, one is by eating food that does not undergo much change in nature.

For example, let's see how many changes the rice we eat has undergone.

1. Wash the rice before cooking it. Washing means removing some dirt by squeezing it and washing it to make it white. Any residue between the husk and the rice is completely removed by this washing.

2. The rice is milled to whiten it before it is brought to the cooking stage. In this process, the nutrient form called thiamin is removed. The form of bran that is thus removed has a grainy texture like flour. I belong to the generation that got the experience of collecting it by hand and eating it at a young age. They taste great. The reason for that taste is the micronutrients in it. In the present milled is done as an action. Oil is extracted from the bran which is removed in this process. There is no doubt that this Oil is healthy. But we do not get the Oil taken in this way. This quality Oil is mixed with synthetic toxic chemicals. If full poison is brought into the market the consequences will be disastrous isn't it? so, That is the compromise provision.

3, Dehusking is another step in natural rice. So there is a three-step process before cooking rice. There are four stages in which husking in paddy cannot be avoided. The husk is the protective covering of rice. Fearing that they will eat it even with the husk, the paddy has developed a fine scale-like thorn above the husk. When a baby girl is fed rice paddy, it gets stuck in the intestine, which is unable to accept anything other than milk, and causes death while talking about rice, do we need all the news about female infanticide here? Some may sneer in disbelief.

It is not surprising that such a frown appears when one succumbs to the culture of eating parboiled rice. Well, back to the rice story.

Separating the husk from the paddy is inevitable and should not be avoided. Next, there is no need to remove the bran between the husk and the rice. The only reason for such removal is the desire to eat rice white, other than our obsession with whiteness.

With the increased use of rice, is it possible to remove only the husk by hand using the old model Motar and pestle? The question may arise.

In this age of technology (sorry, I disagree with the use of the term scientific age) where a second can be divided into a thousand, removing the rice from the paddy without removing the bran is a complete process. But as it is less commercially viable, efforts are not made to do so.

The next time you wash the rice, you don't have to scrub and wash it again and again to keep the rice white. ,

Thus avoiding further processing of grains, pulses, nuts, and tubers as much as possible, the nutrients required from them are obtained without deterioration.

For example, baking dosa by soaking wheat directly and baking dosa is more nutritious than mixing dry wheat flour with water and pouring dosa. The micronutrients of wheat are destroyed and wasted in excessive heat during milling into dry flour.

The flour that is milled in such extreme heat (due to the repeated process) passes through the body as mere waste without providing any nutrients to the body.

Without this instinct, we intellectually avoid waste, and in the evening, we remake the Idly eaten in the morning to make it delicious for the tongue and garbage for the body.

Those of us who save twenty rupees from Idly with upma doesn't seem to have any fear of shelling out thousands for medical treatment.

Care must be taken at every stage in the preparation of food consumed in this disease-ridden era.

Apart from cooking homemade food with care, it is better to completely avoid outside food, especially preserved food such as biscuits, crackers, etc.

It is easy to digest if it is cooked with a mild taste without the intensity of flavors. It is also good to avoid greasy gravies. If you eat such food, you can avoid eating the next meal and eat only fruit and juice as a simple meal.

The first step to health is to eat the next meal only after the previous meal has been fully digested.

We have seen in previous chapters the importance of bathing and walking in getting rid of food waste. The most important thing is to eat the next meal after digesting the food.

"No need for medicine to heal your body's pain,

Ate, when the previous was well digested." (942) Valluvan says.

Knowing that the food eaten earlier has been fully digested and released from its proper place, our granny father says that if we give ourselves praise that it is good, there is no need for medicine for this body called yakkai.

"Knowing the food digested well, when hunger prompted thee,

With constant care, the viands choose that well agree." (944) Valluvan.

He says that there is nothing better than eating after being hungry enough to make sure that the stomach is empty, to ensure that the body absorbs nutrients, and dry well.

"With self-denial take the well-selected meal;

So shall thy frame no sudden sickness feel." (945) Valluvan.

He doesn't like it, he says he likes it, but when the consumption is too much, if he refuses to eat enough, he says that life is stronger. Valluvan stands at the pinnacle in the use of language. He should know how to handle food in moderation just as he handles words in moderation. This level can be known only by talking to the body.

It is only when we eat after digestion that the body can absorb all the nutrients from the food. Just as when water falls on dry land, the land absorbs the water.

If you eat more food on top of the food you ate before it is not fully digested, its nutrients are excreted undigested.

Superstition has been taught that if the stomach is empty without anything, the small intestine will secrete acid and become ulcerated. What feels like acid in an empty stomach is the secretion of old waste. The body tries to find a way to get rid of the waste.

Excess alkalinity and salt retention are not acids waiting to digest the next meal. It is absurd to say that the body secretes acid and waits as if the riot were to stir up panic and build up a reserve force. A soul body never creates evil.

When we smell the food with our nose, when we see the food with our eyes, when the urge to eat is stimulated in us, when the buds of the tongue taste the food, when the teeth chew, the digestive glands secrete enzymes according to the nature of the food at different stages.

The saliva secreted in the mouth after seeing food is sour like acid?

It is only because of eating too much after being hungry and not eating for a long time, and especially because of eating food rich in spices, salt, and oil, which are more than the body's tolerance, that the wastes rush out in the form of evil gas when the previous food is digested and hungry.

During that time, you should continue to eat moderately tasty food. Instead, they are told to eat biscuits in between meals.

They also recommend yogurt to avoid the spicy gravy type. The sourness of curd and the hardness of milk products can aggravate the ulcer.

Suitable food for these times is gelled coconut water bald, palmyra palm Or ice apple, drinks made from padam resin and all kinds of grapes. They provide a feeling of fullness in the stomach, provide good nutrients and flush out the accumulated waste quickly.

The pods are cucumbers for eating raw and pumpkins for cooking.

Body weight may decrease slightly when eating until you are very hungry. So there is no risk. Standardizing body weight to height by BMI is completely ridiculous.

Everybody has a normal weight range. Once you get back to that habit of starving, the weight loss will stop.

Those who do hard work cannot go without food. They will not eat because they cannot work even if they eat too much. We should talk about the food of the workers differently.

Do people who have empty stomachs get ulcers? but diabetes is not the disease that is going to affect our country. The disease that has come will be an ulcer? right.

Keep a good thick tamarind broth in a vessel for ten days and the smell from it will be similar to the smell from the mouth of people with ulcers. The parts of the vessel where the broth is stored are corroded. This is what ulcers are.

There is no better way to eliminate the waste of a diseased diet than to go hungry.

Fasting is a key element in natural remedies. Depending on the severity of the disease, they starve them for two days, four days, a week, Or even ten days and give them only fruits, fruit juices, and freshwater as food.

'Langanam parama ausadam' is a medical adage. That means starvation is the best medicine.

Fasting for one day once a month when normally disease-free will improve detoxification health.

Some keep pouring quality coffees for half an hour in the name of fasting. They say they don't eat and eat the Upma. This is also a type of fraud.

If you have cooked for big parties, the work will not flow. They drink coffee or tea because they don't know the taste. It spoils the technique of the taste buds. The tasters can continue their work while drinking the sherbet. Before tasting, chew a piece of cucumber or a piece of coconut chip and taste it to get an accurate sense of the taste.

An effective way to eliminate waste is to eat plenty of natural, non-oven foods and rest for a long time.

In the final stage of naturopathy, they exclude even fruits and give only water to drink. Eventually, that too ceases and the body receives only breath and cosmic energy. At that point, any chronic toxic waste will be flushed out.

To some, this may seem like a dangerous treatment. But is there anything more dangerous than the treatment given by writing and signing that doctors cannot take responsibility for life during surgery?

We are only talking about people who eat something every hour or every two hours. If we are talking about the food of the working people who are deprived of food and left to starve, then we should be directly talking about politics. We should talk about political economy.

Although food, medicine, health, business, power, and politics are related, we are not talking about direct politics here.

IX

Basics of Food

We have seen a few things related to them in previous chapters. In this chapter, we will go into detail about foods only.

Let's see how to eat without any fear or anxiety on this day when people are getting new panic and rumours about food day by day.

Humans have been eating the food that was available in the area where they traditionally lived. In the last five or six centuries wars and conquests increased and the number of new settlements took place in a big way. People were displaced. In this way, the displaced people shared their traditional foods with the natives of the area and adopted the cuisines of the land as their own.

The food culture of people all over the world has been changing rapidly in the last thirty years, as commercial production has increased and the transportation of goods has increased, as food products have flown from one billion to another billion in the world. At this stage, new ideas about food will inevitably appear.

Since the grains, tubers, vegetables, fruits, and hunting animals grown on land have been the food of the local people for ages, their body's genes have adapted themselves according to the traditional diet.

So even though the new foods available in the market are said to be superior, they are more nutritious and tastier, but the amount of nutrients that the people of the new land get from them is low. Many people may also experience digestive problems.

For example, milk made from soybeans is more nutritious and better than cow's milk. Soy milk, soy butter, soy oil, etc. are important in the daily diet of people in China and East Asian countries. But Indians, especially South Indians, who are capable of digesting any hard food, cannot digest soy-based food.

Even a couple of pieces of meal maker (soya based) added to vegetarian biryani can cause severe stomach upset.

Cereals (varieties) Low-yielding cold-zone people who rely on pastures eat more dairy products and meat. Their digestive capacity is designed accordingly. When they come to our country, if they offer the highest quality rye and ragi flour, they have to leave the next minute. Their bodies are unlikely to have the ability to digest such small-grain food.

Our tongues drool when we taste the jeera-infused jalebi in a baking shop. A westerner or a person of Chinese descent would be horrified to see the same.

Cold zone air has high humidity. No wonder they have no appetite for watery porridges and porridges, the nutritious foods of the tropics.

No matter what we do to the people of our land where the air is hot, brat-based food is not common here. No matter how many slices you eat, you are not satisfied.

A Swiss woman who came to study Indian Christianity had conducted a field study in a Christian school near our restaurant in Hosur. During her stay in Bangalore, she managed something in international restaurants.

After coming to Hosur his body did not accept any of our South Indian food. The school administrator came and handed over the girl to me.

The person who came to eat had no faith in my ability. What do you add while standing in the kitchen preparing each ingredient? He asked what it would taste like.

In the end, after all that, she ordered two homemade dosa and chutney without chilli and left.

I also make oil-less dosa. She said she didn't want chilli in the chutney. So I prepared and sent a chutney thinking that adding a clove of medicinal garlic and ginger with coconut would make the spiciness moderate and not bother the body.

As fast as the parcel went, the lady came running with her red tongue hanging far from her face.

She had tears in her eyes as she said, "Because the chutney was white in colour, I thought that there would be no harm."

We are all tongue-twisters for ginger chutney and garlic chutney. But they do not have the power to withstand even a small amount. I have had to face more than ten experiences like this.

Each region boasts that its cuisine is superior and sophisticated.

There are no categories of fashioned food and unfashionable food in food. There is a saying, "one man's nectar is another man's poison."

So food culture is a conglomerate of geography, ecology, and labour.

Oats are popularised by modern medicine and food marketers as a nutritious, easy-to-appetising food. Normally good nutritious food takes extra time to digest. How can oatmeal be a portion of good and nutritious food that makes you hungry within an hour of eating it?

The fiber in oats indeed cleans bowels. For which Odze himself is ashamed to heap praises upon it.

We can't eat as much of our fiber-rich cereal as we can of rice. But our whole grains are rich in micronutrients.

When you eat rice, you get completeness by adding broth and vegetables to compensate for the lack of nutrients. But only gram and onion are sufficient for people who eat small grains. Kodo millet porridge and two curds of chillies alone are sufficient for a day's hard labour on the land.

Roti cooked in Ragi needs no side dish. The taste of dosa, which is baked in millet rice, can be fully appreciated only when eaten as is. The small grains themselves are rich in aroma and taste. They don't need any other flavourings.

Does a wildflower need grooming? A child who kicks his hand and legs and says "Kuvve. Kuvve" in his own language and smells like milk, the locket accessories will be the beauty of it. Similarly, small grains do not require another by-product.

Small grains are not grown like rice which only drinks water. They are fire bells. Yes, solar energy is absorbed. They store solar energy in themselves. That's why they are so delicious.

Another aspect of this is that rainfed small grains cannot be grown with more chemical fertilizers. If you try to do so, the crops will get scorched in the heat due to lack of water. Small grains are not sprayed with pesticides. Hence its nutrients are not chemically degraded.

The modern generation, alienated from the land and nature, finds our traditional small grains difficult to digest. But within a day or two of starting to eat it, the body adapts itself to the grain. The digestive energy pent up in the body cells is agitated and prepares itself to receive the traditional food.

All the troubles the body experiences while trying to make changes in our diet are temporary. The body attempts to adapt itself.

Another important aspect in adapting ourselves to a healthy lifestyle. A healthy diet.

Naturalists divide the foods we eat into three broad categories.

Stored foods such as chocolate biscuits, chips, crackers, and roasted nuts which are packed dry and transported to different areas are called counter food.

This means that the benefit obtained from these foods is less than the energy expended by the body to digest them. What is the profit if you catch only two small fish in one day?

Cooked rice, vegetables, adai, dosa, idli, gravy, soup, etc. are medium food. Even when we eat such foods, our body expends a lot of energy to digest them. However, it has additional benefits.

Fruits, fruit juices, fresh water, sugarcane juice, neera, honey, aval, etc. Which is suitable food. Such foods are easy to digest. The benefits are high.

As far as we are concerned the body needs the energy to digest any food. But when the balance of the body is disturbed, the way to improve the health of the body is to eat more nutritious food in smaller quantities.

Meat is hard to digest. Naturalists' anti-foods classify.

For us, meat is not such a difficult food. Oil added while cooking meat and excessive spices are the ones that cause severe reactions in digestion. They also prevent the benefits that meat provides to our bodies. Especially in high heat, meats that have been infused with oil cause great harm to the body.

Colour compounds and chemical preservatives are increasing day by day in preserved food as opposed to food.

No shepherd listens to such food vendors. They also influence the ruling class. Quality control teams are staffed by food traders. So any low-quality food gets certified and comes to the market. It is the eaters who lose money for money and have to sacrifice the health of the body.

As if the colour mixture and the chemical compound are not enough, they add a chemical compound that gives only the above smell, which does not have any molecular properties of cocoa and coffee beans, in the name of the aroma of cocoa and coffee.

Also, children's food products are often loaded with toxic chemicals that repeatedly stimulate their taste buds. Individual books are not enough to talk about the danger involved.

There is an urgent need for indiscriminate awareness of such protected foods.

Middle cuisine is rapidly deviating from its regional heritage in both composition and preparation.

For example, twenty or thirty years ago, our method of cooking was to break the pulses in a sieve without heating them and make gravy with them. Today the topping is completely removed and the dal is tampered with. Chemicals are also mixed to prevent the dal from spoiling and insects.

The pulses that come in the market in shiny and pretty packets are just a joke. When the dal is inside the packet, why is it necessary to put the dal image on the top? It is because what is inside is a megass that people have to put the picture of dal on and make people confused.

Ok, let's move on to the next step. Even if we boil the above-mentioned megass dal slowly, that is not the case. Put it in the pressure cooker and boil it on high pressure. Overheating the food leaves the remaining nutrients in the pulp.

You can feel the difference by tasting the dal boiled in a clay pot at moderate heat and the dal boiled in the cooker. Whatever gives taste to the tongue is nutritious.

Well, if we left that sambar with this, that is not the case. We also buy unusual masala powder and mix it when we find that someone worthy of our admiration has appeared directly at a remote party and recommended it. How high heat the powders are milled. How long has it been grinding? Could there be some life in it? What nutrients can this sambar provide us?

The digestive organs, tired of searching for their nutrients in this garbage that enters the stomach under the recognition of food, send the garbage called food from themselves to the waste removal organs. Unable to completely expel the excess waste that accumulates at once, the raw organs, which are overwhelmed, turn a part into gas and send it to the outer parts. This causes gas in different parts of the body.

Well then, for those who are asking the question, what do we do?

Our sambar is not even about two hundred years old. Sambar is one of the few good things left behind by the Maratha Saraboji family who ruled Tanjore. Before that, what did our forefathers cook as gravy?

If we go by that research we have to talk about the fact that within a period of the use of chilli pepper, medicinal pepper played an important role in our diet, and that it was not widespread.

So let's just look at healthy cooking.

The mixer is now common in all middle-class families. It is not a difficult process to put the spices we need in a small jar and grind them once every two or three days. Grinding it like that is best for taste and health.

Keep in mind that packet powders milled at high heat are not safe and can have adverse effects. Whether bought in packets or ground at home, using spices sparingly is good for health. The predominance of spices in our food has increased to such an extent that the face of the raw materials has been destroyed since spices are added as good for digestion.

There is a proverb in our villages that says "keep on washing the baby dissolved " which is the story of Masala.

Next, we can't think of anything other than sambar cooked with pigeon peas. More than that, you can cook broths in various flavours with cowpea, fava beans, which provide good protein content and additional micronutrients, and black chickpeas.

A lot of blame has been placed on coconut for its fat content. Coconut is not high in fat and the fat argument is meaningless. Malayalis, Malaysians, Indonesians and Sri Lankans eat more coconut than Tamils. But how is it that they have fewer heart-related diseases than us as commercial medicine says? And a recent study says that there is no fat in coconuts. This is how analysts report something back and forth.

We should never look at what the papers say. Introspect how you feel after eating any food.

What is the immediate effect? We need to define our diet accordingly, after taking care that certain food is fully digested. No one can recommend a suitable diet for everybody.

Coconut's protein content is moderate and easier to digest than pulses. Rich in nutrients. Can give skin texture.

Another easy alternative to pigeon peas is algae. Sambar can be cooked with split and unpeeled lentils. Wherever chickpea flour is used, algae flour can be used. Especially in making desserts.

While cooking the vegetables, instead of cooking them in oil for a long time, the method of steaming the vegetables in low heat is suitable for health.

Idli, Dosa, and Chapati are the only three types that circulate in the morning and evening under the name breakfast and supper.

In this, we can change small grain Pongal, Idli, Dosa, etc. as our food. Apart from Idli and Dosa, porridge should also be brought to an important place in our cooking. Puttu(which consists of coarsely ground rice, grated coconut, a little salt, and water) is a good bowel cleanser. Today's generation doesn't look haven't look for Puttu.

A small grain porridge or a large porridge cooked with rice will give the body a boost. Urad porridge should be included at least one day a week. Adding urad dal and fenugreek seeds to your morning or evening meal is ideal for health promotion.

Making sure to include spinach two to three days a week is an important step in health. Greens are rich in micronutrients and can increase red blood cell count.

When rice aval and small grain aval are included in the cooking, the cooking is done easily. Her ingredients are suitable for lunch boxes once school children are used to them. It also gives health. Children do not become zombies in schools.

Fruits should be eaten as a one-time meal rather than as an occasional snack. In general, you should give up the habit of buying junk food in packets and bring it home and make it a habit to buy fruits.

Take care of the body after eating food, porridge etc. and you will get a feeling of freedom.

Bringing various foods and flavours like sambar, rasam, red broth (karakkulambu), Veglentil (is a lentil and vegetable stew in South Indian), Vegfries, flatbread, curd, and dessert in lunch at the same time and stuffing it in the stomach will create a huge digestive problem.

Avoiding dairy products completely is best for health. Pickles should also be completely avoided.

Salt, milk, and sugar are called white poison by naturalists. Much of it is true, but there is no need to ignore it with as much fervour as they do.

But by avoiding salt, milk, and sugar when the body is sick, it can recover from the disease quickly.

Similarly, the opposite food should be completely avoided during illness. It is also better to avoid cooked food. If we eat only fruits and fruit juices instead, we can recover from any disease very quickly.

There is no harm in not following the diet we recommend here. But the most important thing to note is that the next meal should be taken only after the previous meal is completely digested.

We have discussed this in detail in the previous chapter.

The next important thing we should consider is diet. The stomach is an elastic, expandable balloon-like bag. Therefore, after each meal, there is room to eat a little more than the amount eaten before. So we cannot judge the stomach capacity properly while eating while sitting on a chair.

We can avoid overeating by sitting on the floor and bending down to eat. If you can't bend down and take the next bite easily, your stomach is full. It can be understood that the limit has been reached.

Next, when we have eaten enough, we have to get up when the wrapped knees start to go numb.

After that, even a small morsel of food becomes a nuisance and a disease.

Many of us understand hunger as the feeling of a slightly empty stomach.

Many of us think of hunger as the feeling of an empty stomach and the feeling of recovery from lethargy after eating when the watery and gelatinous things are easily digested after the stomach is tight. That is, many people consider hunger to be the empty state of the stomach and the emptiness in the stomach. Snacks and drinks like coffee and tea are served between meals.

Starvation is the name for the condition where you can no longer do anything but eat. After reaching that stage, the food eaten is completely digested. Also, all the micronutrients in the food will be absorbed. If we adopt such a habit of eating, our health will not deteriorate.

The fact that food is a medium of energy is being forgotten and the idea that it is a celebration is prevailing among today's generation. We are witnessing a generation that will quickly fall ill without knowing how to measure the level of celebration.

It should be eaten after kneading it well with your hands. This has two advantages. By kneading one we ease the work of grinding in the mouth. When two foods are kneaded in the palm, digestive juices begin to be secreted according to the taste of the kneaded food. Digestion is coordinated by the body.

When we eat with a spoon, our digestion is not fully revealed.

In cold regions, sitting on the cold floor and dipping our hands in cold water before and after eating, we consider it fashionable to eat.

Do you drink water while eating? Drink after eating? They continue to talk about various ideas like how many liters to drink a day, how to drink one liter of water in the morning and how healthy the body is.

All bodies are not created equal. So it is unnatural to standardize it in any aspect.

Generally, the food we eat is watery. So it is not mandatory to drink water while eating or after eating. Depending on the need for food, the body will ask for and receive water. We don't need to pay special attention to it.

Drinking water on an empty stomach half an hour or twenty minutes before a meal prepares the stomach and digestive organs for food. Tamil forefathers have also expressed the same opinion.

Is it necessary to drink a liter of water when you wake up in the morning?

From early morning to midnight, our liver, spleen, kidneys, and other vital organs are actively excreting the previous day's accumulated waste from the body. Early in the morning, the organs and the whole body get rid of dead cells and produce new cells.

In the morning they slowly returned to normal. Drinking a liter of water suddenly in this condition gives a sudden heavy workload to the kidneys and other organs. The workload we put on the body by drinking water in a work environment where the body is not fully prepared for movement can throw the body into confusion.

There is no benefit from drinking this water apart from the fact that the stools come out in a hurry. It also creates fatigue. Some people feel vomiting while drinking water. Vomiting is the counter-feeling at which point anything violently internalized is unnatural.

So can we drink coffee or tea?

As mentioned earlier, when the internal organs are relaxed, it is not appropriate to drink coffee and tea containing milk, which is hotter than the body heat and causes sluggishness.

So what can you drink in the morning?

There is no compulsion to drink anything when you wake up in the morning. If the waste accumulated in the body the previous day has been properly expelled, the body will be naturally active. In this case, you can have breakfast directly after completing the morning exercises and walking.

It is our habitual thinking to drink something before eating. It is not a need of the body. We should get rid of habits that are not good for the body. From the beginning of this book, we have been emphasizing that following what the body tells us is the key to health.

Despite all this, cucumber juice is suitable for those who want something to drink in the morning. Highly nutritious. At the same time, cucumber is rich in micronutrients. Grate about half a cucumber and add water and grind it in a mixer and strain the juice and drink it. It also relaxes the body.

Similarly, another drink is honey water. Mixing one tablespoon of honey with about two hundred ml of water and drinking it will also give health to the body. It also gives good agility.

We have outlined common diets here. Having dinner before seven o'clock and going to bed with an empty stomach and complete digestion of the food eaten is ideal for health. When you turn this into practice, it may seem difficult at first, but it will get easier with time.

You can experience a state of trance during sleep and a refreshing awakening in the morning. People who are used to sleeping with an empty stomach at night will not get sick for the rest of their life.

Food is eaten before 7 o'clock is also just fruit food which will give better health.

We keep on eating because the food we eat is not fully digested. Food is in demand. We eat more than we need.

There is no need to talk about the amount of food that laborers eat. But those whose attention is directed towards labour do not care about food. Usually, people who do brain work tend to overeat. The problem arises because what they eat is not burned.

No one can define this as the amount to eat. Everyone should pay attention to the whole body without looking at the stomach to see if they are full when they eat. Our focus should not be elsewhere. If it is only on the body, the taste of the food will start to decrease. Bored mouth. Stopping eating at this stage is the right measure.

Snacks eaten at meal time are tasty to the tongue but burdensome to the body. Even if you eat as it is, you should reduce the amount of food accordingly. If we eat a small snack or a drink at a certain time today, the way to maintain health is to control the body's habit of wanting to eat something at the same time tomorrow. Control is not minded suppression. Instead, talk to it and make peace with it.

It is not the food we have never seen before that is right before our eyes to stimulate our appetite. Even so, we've had something better before. There will be no chance to eat this on the remaining day. What if that's the case?

Consuming again and again, can we make the body disease and become paralyzed? Human birth itself has a sign of manifesting a superior personality with a healthy body and healthy thinking.

X

A few words about the use of fridge

Many of the middle class have become extravagant spenders. But on the other hand, they are unnecessarily miserly and do not waste food. As a result of this old Indian attitude, they spend all their money on medicine. They do it as a pious thing.

A week's worth of idli, dosa is dough and stored in a fridge, and is taken and eaten now and then. After a day, the dough is tasteless and crumbles.

As we said before, no later food is nutritious. No external changes occur in the Flour, Spinach, and Vegetables kept in the refrigerator. But we do not realize the fact that its life force is destroyed due to climatic changes. That alone gives the food its tastelessness.

It is worse to reheat cooked rice and broth than to eat it as it is. Such food passes through the body as mere food. When we have vegetables within arm's reach, what is the need to stuff them in the fridge?

Women still come to the streets with baskets of vegetables to sell. Then the pushcart comes with onions and tomatoes. As if all this is not enough, the farmers bring home and sell the vegetables. There is no need to buy and store fresh vegetables every day.

Dry flour varieties should be preserved in the refrigerator. We don't protect them that way. After the worm climbs, it is used by boring it with a sieve. If a worm has entered the flour, it means that it has lost its fitness for human consumption.

Dry flours and powders spoil from the minute they are ground. So it stops its gate speed during fridging. It is beneficial to keep dry flour and powder in the fridge.

Keeping the fruit in the fridge from the outside heat may cause it to get cold and shrivel. But when it gets cold, its vital nutrients are destroyed.

Although many people agree with this point of view, because they have bought the fridge, they keep putting something in it out of habit.

The milk harvested in the village is transported to the city. In this itself it undergoes sufficient agitation. Then they pour it into the machine, cool it, separate it, and wash it. Finally, they are cooled and sent to market. It loses its coolness in the outer environment and becomes natural. We buy it and put it back in the fridge. If milk works so hard, what is the vitality we get from it?

From time to time, unable to bear the cat's hungry voice, I buy milk and keep it aside. The cat sniffs eagerly and turns away. Then it comes back. Once touched by the tongue, it runs away. Again, without feeling hungry, he drinks little by little and takes a long time, reluctantly.

We keep the milk that the cat hates and keep it in the fridge in the wild believing that it is rich in calcium.

Cooler boxes can be the best way to protect our products. But never protect our body.

Man has been cooking and eating for at least fifty thousand years. The changes brought about by the older generation with experience in cooking are not harmful to us but beneficial to the body.

But it's the grocers and cookware vendors who are changing our food culture. It is important to approach the cultural changes imposed on us by businessmen and the media with great caution. Food marketers give way to drug marketers. It is not unknown to us that many times drug businesses and food businesses are the same.

Cooking is an art. Each head of the family used to adorn itself with unique art. The health of the entire family was maintained. Each house had its own identity in food taste. But that identity is fading fast. Cooking, which used to be a hobby, has become boring today. Let families become healthier by reclaiming the culinary identity of each family.

XI

When does the cold leave us?

From infancy to the moment when the head hangs down, the cold catches all ages and occasionally shakes it off.

Can't you get relief from the cold?

Funny Vedanta says that "as long as there is a nose, the cold will be". The mucus is not confined to the nose. The mucus is present in every cell of the body. Mucus also transports vital energy from one cell to another (by osmotic diffusion). Phlegm also removes waste from the body.

It was once thought that the human brain was made entirely of mucus. Today they call it fat. This decision may change tomorrow.

Mucus is inexorably abundant in the body. So we can never escape cold.

But when we say that we have a cold, is that cold and the cold in the body the same thing? If you say no, you can say, yes!

Why are you confused?

Cold is always present in our bodies. When the amount of waste accumulated in the body increases to an unbearable level, the body automatically creates a kind of germ and tries to eliminate the waste. when it is held up in the research laboratory and declared to be an axe insect that has come to destroy the clan. It is not an infectious or harmful germ. Good germ.

If the virus comes down to infecting us, there is a chance that we will be infected forever. But it is not contagious.

When the body is weakened, it automatically tries to eliminate waste to maintain its balance. Part of it is mucus discharge.

So why do most people catch colds in the winter or rainy season? The question may arise.

We live in the tropics. Due to internal heat, the removal of waste through the epidermis continues. This procedure is prohibited during monsoons or winters when the humidity in the air increases. As the skin's respiration and elimination of waste are inhibited, the balance of the body is disturbed. To deal with this condition, the body rushes out the unwanted waste products from the body.

During the rainy season, the air we breathe is moist, so the lungs, which separate oxygen and send it to the heart, strive to expel the moist air it has drawn in. It is this effort that drives the sneezing and coughing.

Abundant moist air in the lungs is liquefied and a portion is sent to the colon. Excess water from all these gets mixed in the blood. Then severe body pain occurs. Whether we see medicine or not, the body craves rest. In this case, if you rest, the body heat increases, and suddenly a part of the moisture is expelled.

We try to stop the phlegm by getting annoyed by saying, "rhinorrhea, (I had a runny nose)". They see allopathic medicine. They artificially stimulate the immune system. No effort is completely surrendered. Repeated mucus pushes the body towards rest.

We like the steam. In which the respiratory pores of the skin are opened by steam. Even if you feel free for a while, your body will return to its normal state.

Attempting to expel phlegm, and wateriness is a continuous process. So we should help get it out and not treat it to suppress it. Such treatment only changes the pattern of discharge and does not provide a permanent solution. Such waste can again manifest as a serious disease in another way.

Chronic colds can turn into any disease like body itching, flatulence, tumour, arthritis, high blood pressure, stroke, or heart disease. For such diseases, fat has increased, the knee has worn out, and the heart has become weak. But the reason for this is the phlegm that has accumulated for a long time. No one knows this properly.

So can we never get rid of the effects of cold?

Can. That is what we have seen so far. Simple exercises such as jogging or walking, yoga, etc. should be done regularly to eliminate waste. In cold weather, such exercise helps to increase body temperature and maintain equilibrium.

Next, make it a habit to eat more waste-free foods. Adherence to the holy ritual of bathing. Most important, eat after when you are hungry.

Well, Be that as it may, how do you get rid of colds in winter?

The colon should be kept clean before the onset of winter. Colon cleansing can be done by taking to dysentery Or taking Inima. The colon is the first place where mucus accumulates. If there is no old waste in the colon, the newly formed mucus will take refuge there first, so there will be no immediate harm.

If you start having a cold, if you keep your body warm by jogging, breathing exercises, and doing yoga, the excess moisture accumulated in the body will continue to flow out through moist air.

Next, rest and starvation will be the best medicine. If you starve yourself for a couple of days and rest, you can get rid of a cold that has been bothering you for weeks in just a few days.

Thus we recommend that you avoid cooked food and drink fresh fruit juice. It may seem paradoxical to some because these are diluted foods. But we must understand that these are non-digestible foods. This diluted food should be taken sip by sip and then swallowed after warming it up to body temperature. Drinking like this will not give any adverse effects on the body. Drinking honey from time to time also gives a boost to the body.

There is no need to fear that the body will weaken due to starvation during such treatment. Although it may be weak, the body will return to normal within a day or two after the treatment.

Getting rid of colds and other diseases can lead to better overall health.

We have already seen that the fever in the body at the height of a cold is a waste-burning activity. So if there is a fever we will get relief soon. We can be happy thinking that our bodies will not suffer for some time yet.

XII

There is only one simple solution to all diseases

Whatever disease in the body at any age, in any part, in any form, it is something called waste exposure. Its shapes are different.

Just as we do not panic at the sight of a cold, there is no need to fear spinal cord pain or unexpected cancer. There is only one cure for any disease. It is very simple.

One should cooperate with the body's effort to eliminate waste, i.e. to eliminate the disease, without fear or anxiety. If we do that, we can get rid of the disease completely without any difficulty like surgery, or amputation. Large material costs can be avoided.

Yes, the body itself is always acting as a doctor. The body is capable of bioactive producing chemical elements such as magnesium, phosphorus, potassium, etc., which are necessary for self-healing.

If there is a loss of blood, it will produce an unbelievable amount of blood even if we do not eat.

The body is a sphere. We assume that the liver does only the work of the liver and the spleen only does the work of the spleen.

But it is not true that in the critical phase all the organs are coordinated with each other. That's why when they see positive changes in a body that is weak to the point of death, they are shocked that a "medical miracle" has occurred. The body itself is a miracle.

Even though there are so many sophisticated medical tools, no matter what tests are done on them, some of the diseases that emerge from the body cannot be detected.

A person diagnosed at a young age is hopelessly abandoned by all medicine. They put aside the pessimistic words, "The difficulty is that this person survives and cannot be normal like others who have survived."'

Finally, a person abandoned by his family, without any treatment, without any medicine, suddenly recovers from the disease and becomes a normal human being, and performs unbelievable feats.

Pain during illness is the body's call to life to focus on itself. Whenever pain occurs, if you don't pulsate, moan, and try to stop the pain, the pain will soon disappear. or become a painful ache. The illness will be cured soon.

A person who has been subjected to illness at a young age and has experienced severe pain after overcoming it gains great endurance and resistance and later becomes a person who stands out in society.

So there is no need to fear or feel sorry for the disease. We must understand that illness is a testing ground to increase energy. He who is afraid of disease never leaves him. It makes you dirty and useless. The first step to health is to not fear the disease and dare to face it.

Similarly, during childbirth, they mentally prepare for surgery to escape from the immense pain. One or two children are going to be adopted. Can you fully enjoy the joy of motherhood if you get it through surgery?

I don't look at mothers but ask myself how far the bond between mother and child can be.

There is no doubt that the human species is different from other species. It is a species that knows how to think beyond its food and shelter. For that, he cannot claim to have supernatural powers. If we keep trying to violate nature, it will be bad for man.

A tiny drop of self-control is needed outside this universe. Even those who are conceived to be born to conquer the universe have not been able to escape from surrendering themselves to death in the end.

Living in harmony with nature makes life comfortable. A life that can live without subjecting the body to disturbances such as drugs and treatment will give satisfaction during the lifetime.

Let's live dependent on nature.

We will find fulfillment in life.

Let's complete life.